Health and the State

Volume 187

Series Editor

Lisa Firth

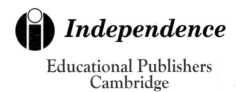 *Independence*

Educational Publishers
Cambridge

First published by Independence
The Studio, High Green
Great Shelford
Cambridge CB22 5EG
England

© Independence 2010

British Library Cataloguing in Publication Data
Health and the State — (Issues ; v.187)
1. Great Britain. National Health Service 2. Medical
policy — Great Britain 3. Public health — Great Britain
I. Series II. Firth, Lisa
362.1'0941-dc22

ISBN-13: 978 1 86168 528 5

Printed in Great Britain
MWL Print Group Ltd

Cover
The illustration on the front cover is by
Simon Kneebone.

CONTENTS

Chapter One: The NHS

Chapter Two: Healthcare Problems

Chapter Three: Healthcare Solutions

Useful information for readers

Dear Reader,

Issues: Health and the State

Following the US debate on free healthcare, there has been much discussion of our own National Health Service. Are we lucky to have healthcare which is free at the point of access, or is the NHS riddled with problems such as bureaucracy and overworked staff? How should it be decided which medicines should be free and which shouldn't? Is free healthcare a right, or a privilege? This book looks at the complex relationship between individual health and state-provided healthcare.

The purpose of *Issues*

Health and the State is the one hundred and eighty-seventh volume in the **Issues** series. The aim of this series is to offer up-to-date information about important issues in our world. Whether you are a regular reader or new to the series, we do hope you find this book a useful overview of the many and complex issues involved in the topic.

Titles in the **Issues** series are resource books designed to be of especial use to those undertaking project work or requiring an overview of facts, opinions and information on a particular subject, particularly as a prelude to undertaking their own research.

The information in this book is not from a single author, publication or organisation; the value of this unique series lies in the fact that it presents information from a wide variety of sources, including:
⇨ Government reports and statistics
⇨ Newspaper articles and features
⇨ Information from think-tanks and policy institutes
⇨ Magazine features and surveys
⇨ Website material
⇨ Literature from lobby groups and charitable organisations.*

Critical evaluation

Because the information reprinted here is from a number of different sources, readers should bear in mind the origin of the text and whether the source is likely to have a particular bias or agenda when presenting information (just as they would if undertaking their own research). It is hoped that, as you read about the many aspects of the issues explored in this book, you will critically evaluate the information presented. It is important that you decide whether you are being presented with facts or opinions. Does the writer give a biased or an unbiased report? If an opinion is being expressed, do you agree with the writer?

Health and the State offers a useful starting point for those who need convenient access to information about the many issues involved. However, it is only a starting point. Following each article is a URL to the relevant organisation's website, which you may wish to visit for further information.

Kind regards,

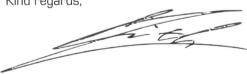

Lisa Firth
Editor, **Issues** series

* Please note that Independence Publishers has no political affiliations or opinions on the topics covered in the Issues series, and any views quoted in this book are not necessarily those of the publisher or its staff.

ISSUES TODAY
A RESOURCE FOR KEY STAGE 3

Younger readers can also benefit from the thorough editorial process which characterises the **Issues** series with our resource books for 11- to 14-year-old students, **Issues Today**. In addition to containing information from a wide range of sources, rewritten with this age group in mind, **Issues Today** titles also feature comprehensive glossaries, an accessible and attractive layout and handy tasks and assignments which can be used in class, for homework or as a revision aid. In addition, these titles are fully photocopiable. For more information, please visit our website (www.independence. co.uk).

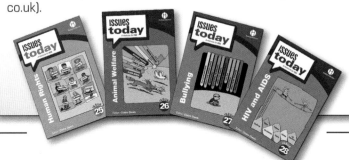

About the NHS – an overview

Since its launch in 1948, the NHS has grown to become the world's largest publicly funded health service. It is also one of the most efficient, most egalitarian and most comprehensive

The NHS was born out of a long-held ideal that good healthcare should be available to all, regardless of wealth. That principle remains at its core. With the exception of charges for some prescriptions and optical and dental services, the NHS remains free at the point of use for anyone who is resident in the UK. That is currently more than 60 million people. It covers everything from antenatal screening and routine treatments for coughs and colds to open heart surgery, accident and emergency treatment and end-of-life care.

Although funded centrally from national taxation, NHS services in England, Northern Ireland, Scotland and Wales are managed separately. While some differences have emerged between these systems in recent years, they remain similar in most respects and continue to be talked about as belonging to a single, unified system.

Scale

The NHS employs more than 1.7 million people. Of those, just under half are clinically qualified, including 120,000 hospital doctors, 40,000 general practitioners (GPs), 400,000 nurses and 25,000 ambulance staff.

Only the Chinese People's Liberation Army, the Wal-Mart supermarket chain and the Indian Railways directly employ more people.

The NHS in England is the biggest part of the system by far, catering to a population of 51 million and employing more than 1.3 million people. The NHS in Scotland, Wales and Northern Ireland employ 165,000, 90,000 and 67,000 people, respectively.

The number of patients using the NHS is equally huge. On average, it deals with one million patients every 36 hours. That's 463 people a minute or almost eight a second. Each week, 700,000 people will visit an NHS dentist, while a further 3,000 will have a heart operation. Each GP in the nation's 10,000-plus practices sees an average of 140 patients a week.

Funding

When the NHS was launched in 1948 it had a budget of £437 million (roughly £9 billion at today's value). In 2008/09 it received over ten times that amount (more than £100 billion).

This equates to an average rise in spending over the full 60-year period of about 4% a year once inflation has been taken into account. However, in recent years investment levels have been double that to fund a major modernisation programme.

Some 60% of the NHS budget is used to pay staff. A further 20% pays for drugs and other supplies, with the remaining 20% split between buildings, equipment and training costs on the one hand and medical equipment, catering and cleaning on the other. Nearly 80% of the total budget is distributed by local trusts in line with the particular health priorities in their areas.

The money to pay for the NHS comes directly from taxation. According to independent bodies such as the King's Fund, this remains the 'cheapest and fairest' way of funding health care when compared with other systems. The 2008/09 budget roughly equates to a contribution of £1,980 for every man, woman and child in the UK.

Structure

The Department of Health controls the NHS. The Secretary of State for Health is the head of the Department of Health and reports to the Prime Minister. The Department of Health controls England's ten Strategic Health Authorities (SHAs), which oversee all NHS activities in England. In turn, each SHA supervises all the NHS trusts in its area. The devolved administrations of Scotland, Wales and Northern Ireland run their local NHS services separately.

Performance

It is difficult to measure the efficiency of healthcare systems. The NHS, like other healthcare systems, has never consistently and systematically measured changes in its patients' health. As a result, it's impossible to say exactly how much the nation's health improves for each pound spent by the NHS.

In the UK, life expectancy has been rising and infant mortality has been falling since the NHS was established. Both figures compare favourably with other nations. Surveys also show that patients are generally satisfied with the care they receive from the NHS. Importantly, people who have had recent direct experience of the NHS tend to report being more satisfied than people who have not.

4 December 2009

⇨ The above information is reprinted with kind permission from NHS Choices. Visit www.nhs.uk for more information on this and other related topics.

© Crown copyright

Private healthcare

Is it always better to cough up and get private treatment? Here's what to expect if you're considering ditching the NHS

What is private healthcare?

Everyone in the UK has a right to free healthcare, provided through the National Health Service (NHS). Some people opt to pay for private medical treatment out of their own pocket. This is known as private healthcare. You can choose to pay for private healthcare through medical insurance, or pay yourself on an ad-hoc basis each time you use private healthcare services.

Why pay for healthcare?

People choose private healthcare for many reasons:

➪ To avoid long NHS waiting lists for specific treatments;

➪ The medical treatment required is not available on the NHS;

➪ The accommodation is more comfortable and often includes an en suite bedroom and TV;

➪ Nursing care, operating theatre and intensive care treatment are included.

Going private might seem more lavish than toughing it out on a no-frills NHS ward, but there are drawbacks

Normally you can choose the hospital and specialist that treats you. Expenses are covered for overnight stays or longer (in-patient coverage) and day-patient coverage (day stays hospital).

So where's the catch?

Going private might seem more lavish than toughing it out on a no-frills NHS ward, but there are drawbacks:

➪ Private medical insurance only covers curable, short-term illness or injury, so inevitably some

By Mariam Manneh

illnesses or treatments will never be covered;

➪ A standard or basic scheme should cover in-patient/daycare treatment, emergency dental work and pregnancy complications, but won't normally cover routine maternity or dental costs.

Many common conditions are not covered by private medical insurance. These include:

➪ Self-inflicted states – drug abuse, self-inflicted injury, normal pregnancy and injuries arising from high-risk hobbies;

➪ Kidney dialysis, organ transplant, gender reassignment, cosmetic and fertility treatment, outpatient medication and dressings.

Patient rights

Most private healthcare insurers now strongly recommend you call their helplines before embarking on a course of treatment and incurring costs. Most insurers provide a client pack, which includes an insurance certificate, claims forms and a helpline card with relevant contact numbers listed. Costs for outpatient treatment can be redeemed through claims forms.

How much information will I have to disclose?

When applying for medical insurance you can opt for medical history declaration cover, or moratorium cover. To obtain medical history declaration cover you will need to fill out a form detailing your medical history. Moratorium cover does not require a medical, but the insurance company may decide not to cover any existing medical condition spanning the last two to five years.

So how much does it all cost?

Any plan agreed between you and a medical insurer should suit your

individual needs, so prices vary a lot from plan to plan. As a rough average, private medical insurance works out at £1,000 per year. You will often be offered a choice between basic, medium and advanced healthcare plans. On minimum cover you can expect to pay around £40 to £50 per month, medium plans average £50 to £60 per month, and advanced plans can cost anything upwards of £65 each month.

As you'd expect, the pricier plans generally cover all health costs for major or minor operations, whereas on a cheaper health plan you may have to absorb up to 50% of treatment costs yourself, or reclaim any money you are entitled to through the claims form process.

Can I get it through work?

Many employers offer their staff the option of private healthcare through reputable private medical care organisations. The employer usually pays for the cost of a corporate medical care scheme. Your employer's HR department or intranet should be able to tell you what options and services are available.

Going abroad for treatment

With private healthcare in the UK often costing more than most of us can afford, a growing number of Brits are heading for sunnier climes to get their treatment abroad.

Routine dental treatments in France, such as fillings and crown replacements, are cheap procedures when compared to UK rates and cost well under £100. Most cosmetic breast surgeries are up to £2,000 cheaper on the Continent, particularly in Spain and Germany.

➪ The above information is reprinted with kind permission from TheSite. org. Please visit www.thesite.org. for more information.

Key statistics on the NHS

Information from the NHS Confederation

NHS funding

⇨ NHS net expenditure has increased from £34.66 billion in 1997/98 to £89.57 billion in 2007/08. Planned net expenditure for 2008/09 is £96.21 billion.

⇨ The money spent by the Department of Health on health services in England per head has risen from £1,165.20 in 2003/04 to a planned £1,717.10 in 2008/09.

⇨ The NHS surplus for the 2007/08 financial year (excluding FTs) was £2.065 billion. The gross deficit for the year was £122 million.

⇨ In 2006/07 the NHS ended the financial year with a net surplus of £526 million. Across the NHS the gross deficit was £917 million, which is down from £1.3 billion for 2005/06.

⇨ Of the extra NHS funding in 2005/06: 52 per cent was spent on higher pay costs; 17 per cent on extra drug costs; seven per cent on capital costs and 13 per cent on more activity and improvements.

⇨ Further analysis from the King's Fund for 2006/07 has estimated that 40 per cent of the additional funding was used for pay and a further 32 per cent was consumed by higher prices and costs associated with NICE recommendations, clinical negligence and capital costs.

NHS organisations

In the NHS there are:

⇨ 172 Acute Trusts (including 82 Foundation Trusts);

⇨ 152 Primary Care Trusts (PCTs);

⇨ 74 Mental Health Trusts (including 32 Foundation Trusts and 16 PCTs providing MH services);

⇨ 12 Ambulance Trusts (including one PCT);

⇨ Ten Strategic Health Authorities;

⇨ Ten Care Trusts (including two PCTs and three MH Trusts) – Care Trusts work in both health and social care and are established when the NHS agrees to work in partnership with local authorities to provide services;

⇨ c.10,500 GP practices in the UK.

NB: some trusts/PCTs are counted twice or more – for example, PCTs providing mental health services or ambulance services.

NHS staff

⇨ The NHS currently employs 133,662 doctors, 408,160 qualified nursing staff, and 39,913 managers.

⇨ The number of doctors employed by the NHS has increased by an annual average of 3.8 per cent since 1998.

⇨ There were more than 41,800 additional doctors employed in the NHS in 2008 compared to 1998.

⇨ There were 84,700 more NHS nurses in 2008 compared to ten years earlier.

⇨ 2,200 more practice nurses were employed by GPs in 2008 than in 2001.

⇨ 51 per cent of NHS employees are Professionally Qualified Clinical Staff.

⇨ Since 2000 the number of front-line staff within the NHS has risen by almost 27 per cent. This rise includes an increase in doctors of 37 per cent; a rise in the number of nurses of 21 per cent; and 18 per cent more ambulance staff.

⇨ Medical school intake rose from 3,749 in 1999/2000 to 6,326 in 2004/05 – a rise of 69 per cent.

⇨ Between 1999/2000 and 2005/06 the number of NHS commissions of pre-registration nurses training increased by 31 per cent.

Management

⇨ Managers and senior managers accounted for 2.9 per cent of the 1.3 million staff employed by the NHS in 2007.

⇨ Between 1998 and 2008 the NHS has recruited 17,220 additional managers, an average annual increase of 5.8 per cent. In the same period more than 126,000 additional doctors and nurses have been recruited.

⇨ In 2007/08 the management costs of the NHS had fallen from five per cent in 1997/98 to three per cent.

⇨ While the NHS spends three per cent of its budget on management costs, equivalent figures for hospitals in Canada and the USA are ten per cent and 17 per cent, respectively.

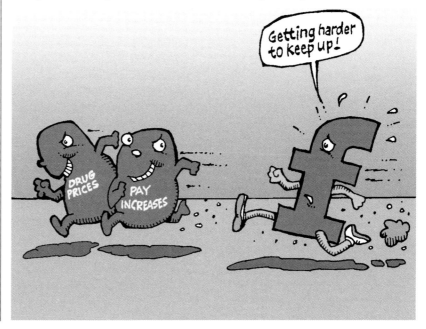

⇨ NHS chief executives' counterparts in the private sector are paid, on average, £424,000 - around three times the average salary within the NHS.

⇨ 32 per cent of NHS chief executives come from a clinical background and over 50 per cent of NHS managers have a clinical background.

⇨ 59 per cent of managers and senior managers in the NHS are female and ten per cent are from minority ethnic groups.

International comparisons

⇨ In comparison with the healthcare systems of five other countries (Australia, Canada, Germany, New Zealand and USA) the NHS was found the most impressive overall by the Commonwealth Fund in 2007.

⇨ The NHS was rated as the best system in terms of quality of care, co-ordination of care, efficiency of care and equity. It was also ranked second behind the USA in relation to the provision of the right form of care and second behind Germany with regards to the provision of safe care.

⇨ In the categories of patient-centred care and access, the NHS was placed fourth. In relation to the maintenance of healthy lives, the NHS ranked equal fourth.

Quality of patient care

⇨ In the 2007 Healthcare Commission inpatient satisfaction survey 92 per cent of the 76,000 respondents rated the care that they received as excellent (42.7 per cent), very good (34.9 per cent) or good (14.3 per cent).

⇨ 78 per cent felt that they were always treated with dignity and respect while using inpatient services.

⇨ 93 per cent said that their room or ward was 'very clean' or 'fairly clean'.

⇨ In the 2005 Healthcare Commission outpatient survey, 93 per cent of people using outpatient services reported their care as being excellent (37 per cent), very good (41 per cent) or good (16 per cent).

⇨ Some 87 per cent of people agreed that they were treated with dignity and respect at all these times while visiting outpatient services.

⇨ 92 per cent of people agreed that their GP always treated them with dignity and respect.

⇨ 96.4 per cent of patients are seen and treated within four hours in A&E.

⇨ 77.1 per cent of category A ambulance calls were responded to within eight minutes in 2007/08 as against a Government target of 75 per cent. This compares with 74.6 per cent in the previous year.

⇨ In 2006/07 the average length of stay in hospital decreased to 6.3 days, compared to 6.9 days the previous year.

The NHS deals with over one million patients every 36 hours

⇨ The median waiting times at the end of February 2009 in England were 2.4 weeks for outpatients and 4.2 weeks for inpatients.

⇨ The number of people waiting longer than six months for treatment as a hospital inpatient fell from 275,460 in April 2000 to 151 by the end of February 2009.

NHS activity

⇨ The NHS deals with over one million patients every 36 hours.

⇨ In 2007/08 there were 1.707 million more elective (planned) admissions than 1997/98.

⇨ In the last ten years the number of emergency incidents attended by ambulance services has doubled to 7.23 million.

⇨ There were almost 88,000 more cataract operations carried out in the NHS in England in 2006/07 compared to 1998/99.

⇨ In 2006/07 the number of heart operations undertaken within the NHS in England had more than doubled since 1998/99 from 40,999 to 81,392.

⇨ Since 1997, 55 new hospital building projects with a value of £30 million or above have been completed. This is the largest ever hospital building programme.

⇨ Between 2003/04 and 2005/06, visits to walk-in centres have increased by 59 per cent to more than 2.5 million, and the number of households receiving intensive homecare has risen by 12.7 per cent.

Health and population

⇨ Life expectancy for men: 77.2 years. Life expectancy for women: 81.5 years.

⇨ The UK population is projected to increase from an estimated 60.6 million in 2006, to 71.1 million in 2031. This is equivalent to an average annual growth rate of 0.69 per cent, or 17.3 per cent over the 25 years. Based on these estimates, the population will exceed 65 million in 2017.

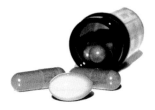

⇨ By 2011 the number of people aged 65 and over is predicted to reach 10,494,000, growing to 15,778,000 by 2031.

⇨ There are an estimated 2.35 million people with diabetes in England and this is predicted to grow to more than 2.5 million by 2010.

⇨ Type 1 diabetes in children is rising at a rate of three per cent a year.

⇨ In England the proportion of men classified as obese increased from 13.2 per cent in 1993 to 23.7 per cent in 2006, and from 16.4 per cent to 24.2 per cent for women over the same timescale.

⇨ In 2002 the direct cost of treating obesity was estimated at between £46–49 million. Between £945 million and £1,075 million was spent on treating the consequences of obesity.

⇨ The above information is reprinted with kind permission from the NHS Confederation. Visit www.nhsconfed. org for more information.

© NHS Confederation

What is the NHS?

The NHS stands for the National Health Service, which provides healthcare for all UK citizens based on their need for healthcare rather than their ability to pay for it. It is funded by taxes

Parliament and Secretary for Health

The Secretary of State for Health is responsible for the work of the Department of Health and reports to the Prime Minister.

The Department of Health is responsible for:
⇨ NHS and social care delivery (through the strategic health authorities);
⇨ systems reform;
⇨ funding and resources;
⇨ strategic communications.

Scotland, Wales, and Northern Ireland run their local NHS services separately.

The following trusts (also called authorities) deliver NHS services on behalf of the Department of Health.

Strategic health authorities (SHAs)

There are ten strategic health authorities in England. On behalf of the Secretary of State, they supervise the trusts in their areas that run NHS services. Their responsibilities include:
⇨ developing plans to improve health services;
⇨ making sure local health services are high quality and perform well;
⇨ integrating national priorities, e.g. improving cancer services, into local health service plans.

Primary care trusts (PCTs)

PCTs provide care when you first have a health problem and need to visit a doctor.

They work with local authorities and health and social care agencies, overseeing 29,000 GPs and 18,000 NHS dentists. There are 152 primary care trusts and they control 80 per cent of the NHS budget.

PCTs make sure there are enough local services for people in their area and that those services are accessible.

By Pamela Brooks, health journalist

PCTs provide:
⇨ hospitals;
⇨ dentists;
⇨ opticians;
⇨ mental health services;
⇨ NHS walk-in centres;
⇨ NHS Direct;
⇨ patient transport, including accident and emergency;
⇨ screening;
⇨ pharmacies.

Acute trusts

Acute trusts manage hospitals to make sure they provide high-quality healthcare and spend money efficiently. They may also:
⇨ decide strategies to develop the hospital and improve services;
⇨ be regional or national centres for more specialised care;
⇨ train health professionals at universities;
⇨ provide services in the community, e.g. health centres, clinics or care at home.

Hospital trusts and foundation trusts

There are 290 NHS hospital trusts that oversee 1,600 NHS hospitals and specialist care centres.

There are also 83 foundation trusts. These are a new type of NHS hospital, run by local managers, staff and members of the public, and are tailored to local needs.

Ambulance trusts

These provide emergency access to health care. There are 13 ambulance trusts in England. Scotland, Wales and Northern Ireland have separate ambulance services.

There are 290 NHS hospital trusts that oversee 1,600 NHS hospitals and specialist care centres

---

The emergency control room prioritises calls for an ambulance and decides what kind of response to send. There are:
⇨ category A emergencies – those that are immediately life-threatening;
⇨ category B or C emergencies that are not life-threatening.

The control room may send an ambulance or a rapid-response vehicle, crewed by a paramedic.

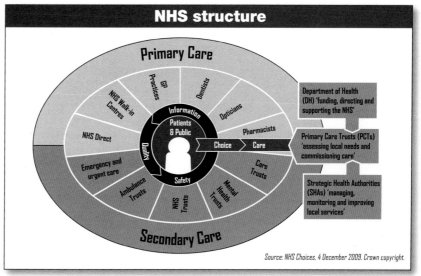

NHS structure

Source: NHS Choices, 4 December 2009. Crown copyright.

Ambulance trusts also provide transport to get patients to hospital for treatment.

Care trusts

These are set up when the NHS and local authorities agree to work together to provide a closer relationship between health and social care.

Their range of services include social care and mental health services.

Special health authorities within the NHS provide a health service to the whole of England or the UK, not just to a local area

---

There are very few care trusts, which are mainly based in England. There are none in Scotland.

Mental health trusts

These provide health and social care services for people with mental health problems.

Services include:
⇨ counselling and psychological therapies;
⇨ community and family support;
⇨ health screening.

They also provide specialist care for people with severe mental health conditions such as severe anxiety problems or psychotic illness.

Special health authorities

Special health authorities within the NHS provide a health service to the whole of England or the UK, not just to a local area. They include the following.

Medicines, Healthcare Products and Regulatory Agency (MHRA)

The MHRA regulates medicines and medical devices in the UK.

It ensures that medicines, healthcare products and medical equipment meet standards of safety, quality, performance and effectiveness and are used safely.

The MRHA grants licences for medicines. It is illegal for companies to sell medicines unless they have a licence.

National Institute for Health and Clinical Excellence (NICE)

NICE provides national guidance on how to promote good health as well as the prevention and treatment of ill health.

It sets guidelines on whether or not certain treatments are available on the NHS in England and Wales.

This guidance is then further assessed by the NHS Quality Improvement Scotland (NHS QIS) and the Department of Health, Social Services and Public Safety in Northern Ireland (DHSSPNI).

National Patient Safety Agency (NPSA)

NPSA has three divisions that help to improve patient safety in the NHS.
⇨ Patient Safety Division (England and Wales) responds to incidents, analyses them and develops action plans. The Scottish Patient Safety Alliance and the DHSSP in Northern Ireland deal with patient safety in those countries.
⇨ National Clinical Assessment Service (UK-wide) gives confidential advice to the NHS when a manager or practitioner is concerned about the performance of a doctor or dentist.

⇨ National Research Ethics Service (UK-wide) promotes ethical research practices to protect the safety, dignity and wellbeing of research participants.

Health Protection Agency (HPA)

The HPA protects the UK against infectious diseases and other dangers to health such as chemical and radiation hazards.

It gives support and advice to the NHS, local authorities, emergency services and Department of Health – including specialist training and carrying out exercises to help prepare the emergency services for major incidents.

It works closely with National Public Health Service Wales, Health Protection Scotland (HPS) and the Department of Health, Social Services and Public Safety, Northern Ireland.

There are three centres.
⇨ Centre for Infections identifies and assesses outbreaks of infectious diseases and monitors vaccine programmes.
⇨ Centre for Radiation, Chemical and Environmental Hazards provides advice to the NHS and other agencies about the health effects of hazards such as chemicals and poisons.
⇨ Centre for Emergency Preparedness and Response coordinates and puts in place strategies for dealing with any release of biological or chemical agents.

10 December 2008

⇨ The above information is reprinted with kind permission from NetDoctor. Visit www.netdoctor.co.uk for more information.

© NetDoctor

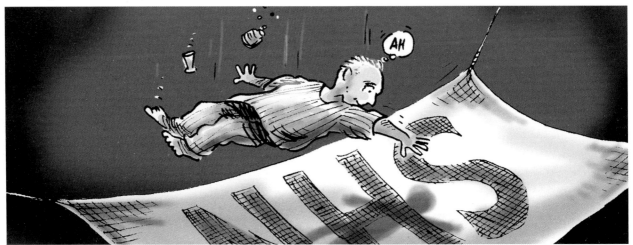

The changing health service

By Dr Ian Greener, Reader in the School of Applied Social Sciences, Durham University, and a researcher within the ESRC's Culture of Consumption Programme

How has the NHS changed over the last 60 years? There have been a number of dramatic improvements in technology so that, from the situation that existed upon the NHS's founding, where GPs had in practice very few treatments that could offer much relief from commonplace illnesses, they can now prescribe a bewildering range of drugs.

There have been rapid growths in medical specialisms and innovations, such as day-surgery, that have elevated skills to levels that would have been jaw-dropping to hospital doctors of the 1940s. The overwhelming majority of NHS staff do a remarkable job when the consequences of their having a single bad day could be considerable for their patients.

However, all is not entirely well with the National Health Service. Medicine has lost some of its lustre as improvements in drug treatment and surgery seem to now be marginal, rather than the dramatic changes that were seen in the 1950s and 1960s. Hospitals remain hugely powerful and continue to absorb a disproportionate amount of resources. Antibiotics have gone from being wonder drugs perceived as an easy cure-all for every type of illness to being over-used and in danger of losing their efficacy. Pharmaceutical companies sometimes seem to be trying to sell new treatments even where their benefits over existing treatments no longer seem great – even if their cost often is.

Patients have changed too. We are no longer grateful for the NHS, having forgotten what it was to worry about the cost of seeing a doctor before making an appointment. We now complain about having to wait, and demand personal and attentive services from health professionals. We are encouraged by the Government to consider ourselves as health consumers rather than patients, and to try and drive reform through our choices of GP and hospital.

The worst-case outcome for the NHS is a combination of medicine no longer being regarded as miraculous, of politicians driving up public expectations of health services to unreasonable levels, and the public deciding that they would rather go to a herbal therapist or reiki healer than their GP.

The National Health Service is not perfect, but we must find ways of improving it through critical appreciation, rather than through derogation; we must find ways of breaking through media-led disaffection, and of celebrating the achievements of the Health Service, not only on its 60th anniversary, but every day.

Summer 2008

⇨ Information from the Economic and Social Research Council. Visit www.esrc.ac.uk and www.socialscienceforschools.org.uk for more information.

© ESRC

NHS 60 years on: snails, snow and Matron

Jean Ellis, 66, was a six-year-old TB patient when the NHS dawned. How greatly things have changed, she tells Jacqui Thornton

In July 1948, I was in the Bath and Wessex Orthopaedic Hospital being treated for TB and as a six-year-old I wasn't aware of the advent of the NHS. It is only in retrospect I realise its huge significance.

The year before, I had a swollen knee, which was eventually diagnosed as tuberculosis. (In rare cases, the infection can spread from the lungs to the bone.) I was told to be good and brave because I had to go to hospital.

It was a horrendous winter that year and the snow was thick. The day I arrived, in my grey flannel coat, the glass doors that made up the entire side of the ward were wide open because that was the cure for TB then – fresh air therapy.

There was wood panelling and dark floors, and two rows of single beds for 30 boys and girls aged from five to ten. I was placed in a Bradford Frame [a metal supporting device for patients with diseases of the spine, hip and pelvis that fitted the shape of the body]. You were strapped to the frame from the armpits to the groin.

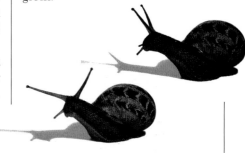

I had no idea what it was supposed to be doing to me. I was on it for months, static day and night. I had a mirror over my bed so I could see people, and to drink I used a feeder with a spout. The nurses used to exercise my good leg and leave my TB leg, which stopped growing.

If only people realised how lucky they are

It was a strict regime; Matron and the sisters ruled. Everything had to be pristine. During the surgeon's ward round, the fear was tangible and we children picked up on it. The surgeons would come to the bed and just say 'right TB knee' – so I almost thought that was my name.

I can't remember anyone who was gentle or kind. My surgeon – unusually, a woman – was the redoubtable Maud Forrester-Brown, who, in the winter, would ski to the hospital, and in the summer came by horse.

Visiting was two Saturdays a month and every other Sunday for two hours. At two o'clock you would hear footsteps on the corridor and you stared at the door waiting. My parents were very affectionate and would bring me comics, but our time together was so brief, it was awful watching them go.

One of my first memories was of a little blond boy in the next bed being sent to have an operation and not coming back. The staff didn't talk about it. Months later, the sister said, 'I have some good news for you', and I thought I was going home, but then she told me I was going to have an operation. I cried dreadfully because I thought I was going to die.

The days were endless: there was no amusement, no toys. We used to race snails to pass the time. The food was austere and served on tin plates – I can't eat steamed fish to this day.

We had sparse tuition, maybe two hours in the morning – I couldn't read until I was nine. My worst memory is my punishment for being untidy. I was taken to the plaster room, away from the wards, with huge casts of torsos and arms and legs. I don't know how long I was left there – it could have been only five minutes – but I remember it being the most frightening experience ever.

I do have some pleasant memories. We had Brownies meetings, with our beds pushed into a circle. November the fifth was another highlight when the Scouts let off fireworks in front of the hospital and one of them would go to the fish shop and get bags of chips for us. (It's still my favourite food.)

At Christmas, the surgeons used to come in to carve the turkey and, once, the nurses were going to a New Year's Eve ball and we begged them to show us their evening dresses. It was amazing seeing these nurses who had plain, boring uniforms suddenly transformed into princesses.

When I was discharged, aged seven, things seemed so small after being in such a big environment. I was astonished by traffic and noise.

It's only really with the 60th anniversary of the NHS that you realise the difference between then and now is so extreme. I have just had a hip replacement; it was an amazing experience. I have been in reception areas of hotels that didn't look as good; the surgeon was so kind and understanding and the staff couldn't do enough.

If only people realised how lucky they are. The care for my age group is outstanding and that's because we have a National Health Service. I shall be eternally grateful for it.
30 June 2008

NHS 60 – health protection timeline

Information from the Health Protection Agency

1940s

1948: The National Health Service is established on 5 July. For the first time hospitals, doctors, nurses, pharmacists and dentists provide services that are free for all at the point of delivery.

1948: Andrew J. Moyer is granted a patent to mass produce penicillin, the antibiotic that was discovered and developed in 1928 by Alexander Fleming. There is already evidence that some bugs are developing a resistance to penicillin, most notably staphylococcus aureus, a bacterium

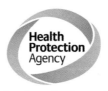

that can live harmlessly on the body, but can cause disease, particularly if there is an opportunity for the bacteria to enter the body.

1948: The results of a controlled UK-wide trial of the TB drug streptomycin are published in October. Within a few years streptomycin will be widely adopted as the treatment of choice against pulmonary TB.

1950s

1950: 50,000 cases of TB are recorded in the UK.

1951: Richard Doll and Austin Bradford Hill publish a paper on a survey they carried out that links smoking and lung cancer for the first time.

1953: BCG vaccination is introduced in secondary schools in the UK. This, combined with the mass X-ray programmes of the 1950s and 1960s, dramatically reduces the number of recorded cases, but TB doesn't disappear entirely.

1954: Doll and Hill establish the link between smoking and lung cancer beyond doubt and publish the evidence. The Government accepts their research findings.

1956: Clean Air Act (see also 1968 and 1993) introduces smokeless zones and regulates stack heights for industries that produce smoke pollution.

1956: Britain's first industrial-scale nuclear power station opens in Calder Hall at Windscale, near Sellafield in West Cumbria.

1957: An accident occurs at the nuclear reactor at Windscale. A report of the Inquiry into the accident is published but some data on the releases are omitted for security reasons. The full facts are not known for 30 years.

1957: Asian flu sweeps the world, causing an estimated two million excess deaths.

1960s

1961: A combined Diphtheria, Tetanus and Pertussis vaccine is introduced. Up to 70,000 cases of diphtheria were recorded in the UK in the 1950s, leading to 5,000 deaths.

1962: A live attenuated polio vaccine introduced. Prior to the introduction of a vaccine, epidemic years would see as many as 8,000 cases of polio in the UK. Today there are no cases of paralysis from polio in this country.

1963: First Nuclear Test Ban Treaty is signed, banning tests in the atmosphere, in space and under water.

1968: The first measles vaccine is introduced to the childhood immunisation programme. 236,154 measles cases were notified that year and 51 children died from the disease.

1968: Another flu pandemic, this time Hong Kong flu. Excess deaths are estimated at one million globally.

1968: Clean Air Act (See 1993)

1970s

1970s: Smoke detectors are gradually introduced to domestic premises over the decade, saving many lives.

1976: Legionnaires' disease, a form of bacterial pneumonia, is recognised for the first time following an outbreak in Philadelphia.

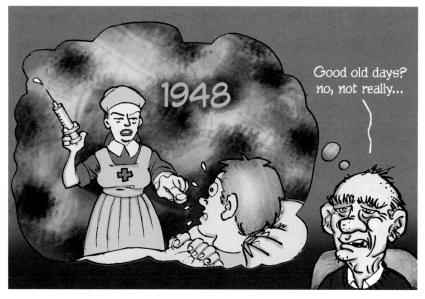

Good old days? no, not really...

1979: Serious nuclear accident at Three Mile Island in the USA. Fortunately its secure containment prevents any significant releases of radioactive material into the environment.

1979: A commission of eminent scientists declares that smallpox has been eradicated from the world.

1980s

1980: The World Health Organization endorses the declaration on smallpox eradication on 8 May. It is estimated that smallpox caused 300–500 million deaths in the 20th century. As recently as 1967, 15 million cases were recorded worldwide and two million people died from the disease.

1981: The first case of AIDS is reported in the UK.

1982: Hepatitis B vaccine is introduced.

1984: The report of an inquiry into a food poisoning outbreak at Stanley Royd Hospital in Wakefield recommends the establishment of Consultant in Communicable Disease Control (CCDC) posts. 300 patients and staff were taken ill in the outbreak and 19 elderly patients died.

1985: HIV testing is introduced in Genitourinary Medicine (GUM) clinics for the first time.

1985: BSE (bovine, spongiform encephalitis) first identified in UK cattle.

1986: The world's worst nuclear power accident occurs at Chernobyl in the Ukraine, then part of the Soviet Union. Radiation monitoring in the UK shows elevated levels due to fallout from the accident.

1987: 5,745 TB cases recorded in the UK, an all-time low. Since then, instances of the disease have slowly but steadily increased to the present level of 8,000 cases a year. TB is usually treatable with antibiotics.

1988: MMR, the measles, mumps and rubella vaccine, is introduced. Before the introduction of MMR vaccine, around 1,200 people were admitted to hospital each year with mumps, meningitis or encephalitis and an average of 50 babies were born with severe rubella damage.

1989: Hepatitis C infection is identified for the first time.

1990s

1993: Clean Air Act of 1993 consolidates previous Clean Air Acts of 1956 and 1968. It prohibits the emission of dark smoke from chimneys, decrees that new furnaces 'shall be so far as is practicable smokeless' and creates smoke-control areas.

1997: The first proven links are made between BSE in cattle and new variant CJD (vCJD) in humans.

1997: Combined Diphtheria, Tetanus and Pertussis (DTP)-Hib vaccine is introduced. Before the introduction of haemophilus influenzae type b (Hib) vaccination, one in every 600 children developed Hib meningitis or other serious forms of disease before their fifth birthday. Today there are only a handful of cases in young children. Tetanus has all but disappeared in UK children.

1998: Uptake of MMR vaccination (Measles, Mumps and Rubella) is affected by reports of 'research' linking the vaccine with autism. Since then, successive studies have proved that MMR is safe and effective and parental confidence in the vaccine is recovering.

The National Health Service was established on 5 July 1948. For the first time hospitals, doctors, nurses, pharmacists and dentists provide services that are free for all at the point of delivery

---

1999: Tobacco advertising is banned in shops and newsagents.

1999: In an initiative to protect unborn babies from infection, HIV testing is offered for the first time to pregnant women as part of their routine antenatal care.

2000s

2000: Leaded petrol banned in the UK, except for use in classic cars.

2000: The Stewart Report on Mobile Phones and Health recommends a precautionary approach to new technology that has become widely used by the public, including children.

2002: First outbreaks of SARS (severe acute respiratory syndrome) occur in Southeast Asia and Canada.

2003: Legislation is introduced to end tobacco sponsorship of sports.

2003: The Health Protection Agency (HPA) is set up in April by bringing together the former Public Health Laboratory Service (PHLS), the national Chemical Hazards and Poisons Division (ChaPD), the microbiological research establishment at Porton Down in Wiltshire and Consultants in Communicable Disease Control and Health Protection Nurses who were formerly employed by Health Authorities in the regions.

2005: The Health Protection Agency is established as a non-departmental public body 'to protect the community (or any part of the community) against infectious diseases and other dangers to health' (HPA Act 2004). The National Radiological Protection Board is assimilated and becomes the Agency's Radiation Protection Division.

2005: The biggest explosion and fire in Europe since World War 2 occurs at the Buncefield oil depot in Hertfordshire. The Health Protection Agency carries out environmental sampling and advises on health precautions, including advice on the potential impact of materials used to extinguish the fire.

2005: The BCG immunisation programme is refined to meet modern needs. The vaccine is now given routinely to babies in areas with TB rates of 40 cases per 100,000 of population or above and to babies who are at greater risk of coming into contact with a TB patient due to family or personal circumstances.

2006: The Pneumococcal Conjugate Vaccine (PCV) is introduced into the childhood immunisation programme in September, preventing an estimated 470 cases of serious illness or death in young children since then.

2006: Alexander Litvinenko dies from radiation poisoning following ingestion of Polonium 210 in November. The Health Protection Agency monitors his family, friends, close associates, hospital staff who treated him and staff in the various hotels, offices and restaurants that he and his associates visited. Environmental checks at various locations provide evidence for HPA staff to give public reassurance on the wider risks to health.

2007: Legislation to ban smoking in workplaces and public premises comes in to effect.

2007: Britain's first H5N1 outbreak in bird flocks occurs at a poultry processing plant in Suffolk. The HPA creates the capability to test suspected H5N1 specimens at laboratories across England, ensuring a rapid response if a human should be suspected of acquiring H5N1 infection.

2007: Summer floods devastate homes and businesses across Yorkshire, Humber and south west England. The HPA provides expert advice on protection from chemical hazards and infectious disease.

2008: HPA and NHS partners prepare for the launch of the Human Papilloma Virus (HPV) vaccination programme, due to be launched in secondary schools in September. It will protect girls from a virus that causes cervical cancer.

2008: The HPA is working with partners on the development of a Meningococcal B vaccine, which should be available within the foreseeable future.

15 July 2008

⇨ The above information is reprinted with kind permission from the Health Protection Agency. Visit www.hpa.org.uk for more information.

© Health Protection Agency

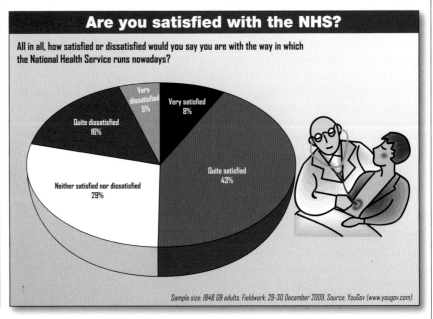

Are you satisfied with the NHS?

All in all, how satisfied or dissatisfied would you say you are with the way in which the National Health Service runs nowadays?

- Very dissatisfied 5%
- Very satisfied 8%
- Quite dissatisfied 16%
- Quite satisfied 43%
- Neither satisfied nor dissatisfied 29%

Sample size: 1848 GB adults. Fieldwork: 29-30 December 2009. Source: YouGov (www.yougov.com)

How healthy are we?

What the Health Profile of England 2008 shows – the general picture

A general improvement in health outcome

The report shows recent improvements in a number of critical areas, e.g.:

⇨ declining mortality rates in targeted killers (cancers, all circulatory diseases and suicides);

⇨ increasing life expectancy, now at its highest ever level;

⇨ reducing infant mortality, now at its lowest ever level.

However, in some areas particular challenges remain to achieve and sustain progress, e.g.:

⇨ rising rates of diabetes;

⇨ rising rates of chlamydia.

Similarly for the determinants of health, although we are making improvements in some important areas, e.g.:

⇨ the number of people who smoke;

⇨ quality of housing stock;

⇨ increases in physical activity levels and fruit and vegetable consumption.

There are areas of concern, e.g.:

⇨ increasing levels of obesity in adults and children (and even where we are seeing improvements, health inequalities are often present);

⇨ the report illustrates various geographical inequalities across the country.

International comparisons give a wider context presenting national progress in comparison to countries of the European Union (EU), or to the 15 countries that were members of the EU prior to 2004 (EU-15), e.g.:

⇨ Premature death rates from all circulatory diseases have shown a narrowing of the gap with the EU-15 average over recent decades, but remain higher than the average for this group.

⇨ Premature mortality rates from cancer for males have, over the last 30 years, fallen substantially faster than the EU-15 average and are now among the lowest in the EU-15; for females, rates which were once substantially higher than the EU-15 average are now rather closer to the EU-15 average.

⇨ Death rates from motor vehicle traffic accidents in the United Kingdom are among the lowest in the EU.

⇨ The prevalence of obesity in England is the highest in the EU-15 countries, and one of the highest in the wider cohort of OECD countries.

⇨ Death rates for chronic liver disease and cirrhosis have risen markedly, particularly since the mid-1990s, and for females, recent data show that England has risen above the EU-15 average.

⇨ The percentage of all live births to mothers under age 20 in the United Kingdom is the highest when compared to other EU-15 countries.

January 2009

⇨ The above information is the executive summary of the *Health Profile of England 2008* report, and is reprinted with kind permission from the Department of Health. Visit their website at www.dh.gov.uk for more information.

The NHS at 60

An online survey of patients' views – executive summary

⇨ The majority of respondents still use the NHS exclusively as their only source of health treatment. 61.1% of those who took part in the survey stated this to be the case with a further 25.5% of people stating that they use both public and private healthcare.

⇨ General Practitioners (GPs) and Consultants remain the first point of reference concerning health matters (50.3%). The Internet was second (22%) as a source of information for patients. This is interesting for those seeking to ensure accurate information reaches patients in the most accessible and acceptable way.

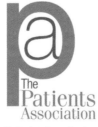

The Patients Association

listening to patients
speaking up for change

⇨ Respondents had concerns about spending on NHS bureaucracy. When asked what they considered a waste, nearly 30% believe non-clinical staff contribute to waste in the NHS. 'Waste by patients' ranked second to this at 24.1%. It was cited by respondents as a significant cause of waste within the NHS. This is particularly interesting and the Patients Association intends to investigate more fully. There are a wide variety of reasons and/or perceptions that could lead to this view.

⇨ We looked at the financing of the NHS from another angle and invited respondents to suggest treatments that should not be covered by the NHS. The highest percentage, 40.9%, opted for cosmetic surgery.

⇨ There is no desire for change in the way healthcare is funded in the UK. 40% of respondents stated that they wanted to continue to pay for their healthcare through general taxation, reflecting convictions that a public and not private health system for all is still necessary.

⇨ A significant amount of respondents (20.5%) stated that en-suite facilities should be charged for within the NHS as a means of providing finance to the service. There was also moderate supporting evidence for levying charges in respect of: access to medical records, communications in hospital and car parking charges, as alternative sources of finance.

⇨ Over 70% said patients must be able to seek financial compensation from the NHS when things go wrong. However, respondents were divided between what form the compensation should take: 34% stated that there should be a standard fixed rate of compensation while 43.6% stated that the compensation should be settled through legal proceedings.

⇨ The strongest view in the entire survey was the 81% wanting to see 'core' levels of service regardless of location, in other words, no postcode lottery. 19% favoured local services decided on the basis of local clinical need.

⇨ There was a high level of response to our question asking about the legal rights of patients to such elements of care as minimum standards, safe environments and second opinions.

⇨ When asked what factor would make the greatest difference to patients in their experience of the NHS in primary care, respondents wanted improved out-of-hours services (50.1%) and dental care (47.4%). In secondary care, 60.1% wanted more hospital staff and reduced hospital acquired infections, e.g. MRSA.

April 2008

⇨ The above information is reprinted with kind permission from the Patients Association. Visit www. patients-association.org.uk for more information.

© *Patients Association*

The NHS Constitution

The NHS belongs to us all

The NHS belongs to the people

It is there to improve our health and well-being, supporting us to keep mentally and physically well, to get better when we are ill and, when we cannot fully recover, to stay as well as we can to the end of our lives. It works at the limits of science - bringing the highest levels of human knowledge and skill to save lives and improve health. It touches our lives at times of basic human need, when care and compassion are what matter most.

The NHS is founded on a common set of principles and values that bind together the communities and people it serves - patients and public - and the staff who work for it.

This Constitution establishes the principles and values of the NHS in England. It sets out rights to which patients, public and staff are entitled, and pledges which the NHS is committed to achieve, together with responsibilities which the public, patients and staff owe to one another to ensure that the NHS operates fairly and effectively. All NHS bodies and private and third sector providers supplying NHS services will be required by law to take account of this Constitution in their decisions and actions.

The Constitution will be renewed every ten years, with the involvement of the public, patients and staff. It will be accompanied by the *Handbook to the NHS Constitution*, to be renewed at least every three years, setting out current guidance on the rights, pledges, duties and responsibilities established by the Constitution. These requirements for renewal will be made legally binding. They will guarantee that the principles and values which underpin the NHS are subject to regular review and recommitment; and that any Government which seeks to alter the principles or values of the NHS, or the rights, pledges, duties and responsibilities set out in this Constitution, will have to engage in a full and transparent debate with the public, patients and staff.

Principles that guide the NHS

Seven key principles guide the NHS in all it does. They are underpinned by core NHS values which have been derived from extensive discussions with staff, patients and the public. These values are set out at the back of this document.

1 The NHS provides a comprehensive service, available to all irrespective of gender, race, disability, age, sexual orientation, religion or belief. It has a duty to each and every individual that it serves and must respect their human rights. At the same time, it has a wider social duty to promote equality through the services it provides and to pay particular attention to groups or sections of society where improvements in health and life expectancy are not keeping pace with the rest of the population.

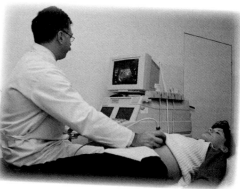

2 Access to NHS services is based on clinical need, not an individual's ability to pay. NHS services are free of charge, except in limited circumstances sanctioned by Parliament.

3 The NHS aspires to the highest standards of excellence and professionalism – in the provision of high-quality care that is safe, effective and focused on patient experience; in the planning and delivery of the clinical and other services it provides; in the people it employs and the education, training and development they receive; in the leadership and management of its organisations; and through its commitment to innovation and to the promotion and conduct of research to improve the current and future health and care of the population.

4 NHS services must reflect the needs and preferences of patients, their families and their carers. Patients, with their families and carers, where appropriate, will be involved in and consulted on all decisions about their care and treatment.

5 The NHS works across organisational boundaries and in partnership with other organisations in the interest of patients, local communities and the wider population. The NHS is an integrated system of organisations and services bound together by the principles and values now reflected in the Constitution. The NHS is committed to working jointly with local authorities and a wide range of other private, public and third sector organisations at national and local level to provide and deliver improvements in health and well-being.

6 The NHS is committed to providing best value for taxpayers' money and the most effective, fair and sustainable use of finite resources. Public funds for healthcare will be devoted solely to the benefit of the people that the NHS serves.

7 The NHS is accountable to the public, communities and patients that it serves. The NHS is a national service funded through national taxation, and it is the Government which sets the framework for the NHS and which is accountable to Parliament for its operation. However, most decisions in the NHS, especially those about

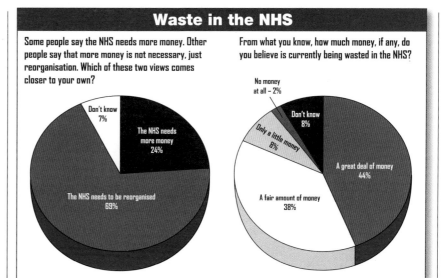

Waste in the NHS

Some people say the NHS needs more money. Other people say that more money is not necessary, just reorganisation. Which of these two views comes closer to your own?

- Don't know 7%
- The NHS needs more money 24%
- The NHS needs to be reorganised 69%

From what you know, how much money, if any, do you believe is currently being wasted in the NHS?

- No money at all – 2%
- Don't know 8%
- Only a little money 8%
- A great deal of money 44%
- A fair amount of money 38%

Sample size: 2163. Fieldwork: 23-25 June 2008. Source: YouGov (www.yougov.com)

the treatment of individuals and the detailed organisation of services, are rightly taken by the local NHS and by patients with their clinicians. The system of responsibility and accountability for taking decisions in the NHS should be transparent and clear to the public, patients and staff. The Government will ensure that there is always a clear and up-to-date statement of NHS accountability for this purpose.

Patients and the public – your rights and NHS pledges to you

Everyone who uses the NHS should understand what legal rights they have. For this reason, important legal rights are summarised in this Constitution and explained in more detail in the *Handbook to the NHS Constitution*, which also explains what you can do if you think you have not received what is rightfully yours. This summary does not alter the content of your legal rights.

The Constitution also contains pledges that the NHS is committed to achieve. Pledges go above and beyond legal rights. This means that pledges are not legally binding but represent a commitment by the NHS to provide high-quality services.

Access to health services:

You have the right to receive NHS services free of charge, apart from certain limited exceptions sanctioned by Parliament.

You have the right to access NHS services. You will not be refused access on unreasonable grounds.

You have the right to expect your local NHS to assess the health requirements of the local community and to commission and put in place the services to meet those needs as considered necessary.

You have the right, in certain circumstances, to go to other European Economic Area countries or Switzerland for treatment which would be available to you through your NHS commissioner.

You have the right not to be unlawfully discriminated against in the provision of NHS services including on grounds of gender, race, religion or belief, sexual orientation, disability (including learning disability or mental illness) or age.[1]

The NHS also commits:

⇨ to provide convenient, easy access to services within the waiting times set out in the *Handbook to the NHS Constitution* (pledge);

⇨ to make decisions in a clear and transparent way, so that patients and the public can understand how services are planned and delivered (pledge); and

⇨ to make the transition as smooth as possible when you are referred between services, and to include you in relevant discussions (pledge).

Quality of care and environment:

You have the right to be treated with a professional standard of care, by appropriately qualified and experienced staff, in a properly approved or registered organisation that meets required levels of safety and quality.[2]

You have the right to expect NHS organisations to monitor, and make efforts to improve, the quality of healthcare they commission or provide.

The NHS also commits:

⇨ to ensure that services are provided in a clean and safe environment that is fit for purpose, based on national best practice (pledge); and

⇨ to continuous improvement in the quality of services you receive, identifying and sharing best practice in quality of care and treatments (pledge).

Everyone who uses the NHS should understand what legal rights they have

---

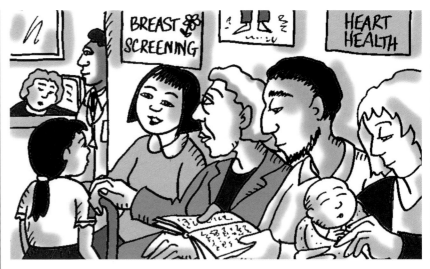

Nationally approved treatments, drugs and programmes:

You have the right to drugs and treatments that have been recommended by NICE[3] for use in the NHS, if your doctor says they are clinically appropriate for you.

You have the right to expect local decisions on funding of other drugs and treatments to be made rationally following a proper consideration of the evidence. If the local NHS decides not to fund a drug or treatment you and your doctor feel would be right for you, they will explain that decision to you.

You have the right to receive the vaccinations that the Joint Committee on Vaccination and Immunisation recommends that you should receive under an NHS-provided national immunisation programme.

The NHS also commits:

⇨ to provide screening programmes as recommended by the UK National Screening Committee (pledge).

Respect, consent and confidentiality:

You have the right to be treated with dignity and respect, in accordance with your human rights.

You have the right to accept or refuse treatment that is offered to you, and not to be given any physical examination or treatment unless you have given valid consent. If you do not have the capacity to do so, consent must be obtained from a person legally able to act on your behalf, or the treatment must be in your best interests.[4]

Patients and the public – your rights and NHS pledges to you:

You have the right to be given information about your proposed treatment in advance, including any significant risks and any alternative treatments which may be available, and the risks involved in doing nothing.

You have the right to privacy and confidentiality and to expect the NHS to keep your confidential information safe and secure.

You have the right of access to your own health records. These will always be used to manage your treatment in your best interests.

The NHS also commits:

⇨ to share with you any letters sent between clinicians about your care (pledge).

Informed choice:

You have the right to choose your GP practice, and to be accepted by that practice unless there are reasonable grounds to refuse, in which case you will be informed of those reasons.

You have the right to express a preference for using a particular doctor within your GP practice, and for the practice to try to comply.

You have the right to make choices about your NHS care and to information to support these choices. The options available to you will develop over time and depend on your individual needs. Details are set out in the *Handbook to the NHS Constitution.*

The NHS also commits:

⇨ to inform you about the healthcare services available to you, locally and nationally (pledge); and

⇨ to offer you easily accessible, reliable and relevant information to enable you to participate fully in your own healthcare decisions and to support you in making choices. This will include information on the quality of clinical services where there is robust and accurate information available (pledge).

Involvement in your healthcare and in the NHS:

You have the right to be involved in discussions and decisions about your healthcare, and to be given information to enable you to do this.

You have the right to be involved, directly or through representatives, in the planning of healthcare services, the development and consideration of proposals for changes in the way those services are provided, and in decisions to be made affecting the operation of those services.

The NHS also commits:

⇨ to provide you with the information you need to influence and scrutinise the planning and delivery of NHS services (pledge); and

⇨ to work in partnership with you, your family, carers and representatives (pledge).

Complaint and redress:

You have the right to have any complaint you make about NHS services dealt with efficiently and to have it properly investigated.

You have the right to know the outcome of any investigation into your complaint.

You have the right to take your complaint to the independent Health Service Ombudsman, if you are not satisfied with the way your complaint has been dealt with by the NHS.

You have the right to make a claim for judicial review if you think you have been directly affected by an unlawful act or decision of an NHS body.

You have the right to compensation where you have been harmed by negligent treatment.

The NHS also commits:

⇨ to ensure you are treated with courtesy and you receive appropriate support throughout the handling of a complaint; and the fact that you have complained will not adversely affect your future treatment (pledge);

⇨ when mistakes happen, to acknowledge them, apologise, explain what went wrong and put things right quickly and effectively (pledge); and

⇨ to ensure that the organisation learns lessons from complaints and claims and uses these to improve NHS services (pledge).

Patients and the public – your responsibilities

The NHS belongs to all of us. There are things that we can all do for ourselves and for one another to help it work effectively, and to ensure resources are used responsibly.

You should recognise that you can make a significant contribution to your own, and your family's, good health and well-being, and take some personal responsibility for it.

You should register with a GP practice – the main point of access to NHS care.

You should treat NHS staff and other patients with respect and recognise that causing a nuisance or disturbance on NHS premises could result in prosecution.

You should provide accurate information about your health, condition and status.

You should keep appointments, or cancel within reasonable time. Receiving treatment within the maximum waiting times may be compromised unless you do.

You should follow the course of treatment which you have agreed, and talk to your clinician if you find this difficult.

You should participate in important public health programmes such as vaccination.

You should ensure that those closest to you are aware of your wishes about organ donation.

You should give feedback – both positive and negative – about the treatment and care you have received, including any adverse reactions you may have had.

Notes

1 The Government intends to use the Equality Bill to make unjustifiable age discrimination against adults unlawful in the provision of services and exercise of public functions. Subject to Parliamentary approval, this right not to be discriminated against will extend to age when the relevant provisions are brought into force for the health sector.

2 The registration system will apply to some NHS providers in respect of infection control from 2009, and more broadly from 2010. Further detail is set out in the *Handbook to the NHS Constitution*.

3 NICE (the National Institute for Health and Clinical Excellence) is an independent NHS organisation producing guidance on drugs and treatments. 'Recommended' means recommended by a NICE technology appraisal. Primary care trusts are normally obliged to fund NICE technology appraisals from a date no later than three months from the publication of the appraisal.

4 If you are detained in hospital or on supervised community treatment under the Mental Health Act 1983, different rules may apply to treatment for your mental disorder. These rules will be explained to you at the time. They may mean that you can be given treatment for your mental disorder even though you do not consent.

21 January 2009

⇨ The above information is an extract from the NHS Constitution for England and is reprinted with kind permission from the Department of Health. Please visit www.dh.gov.uk for more information.

© Crown copyright

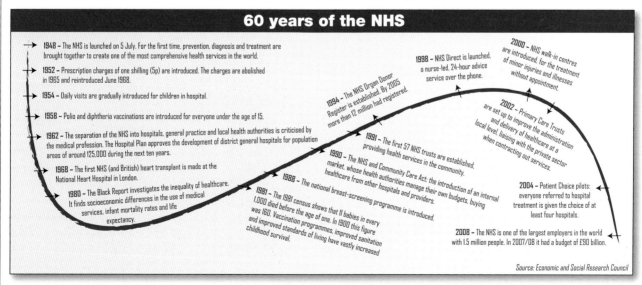

60 years of the NHS

1948 – The NHS is launched on 5 July. For the first time, prevention, diagnosis and treatment are brought together to create one of the most comprehensive health services in the world.

1952 – Prescription charges of one shilling (5p) are introduced. The charges are abolished in 1965 and reintroduced June 1968.

1954 – Daily visits are gradually introduced for children in hospital.

1958 – Polio and diphtheria vaccinations are introduced for everyone under the age of 15.

1962 – The separation of the NHS into hospitals, general practice and local health authorities is criticised by the medical profession. The Hospital Plan approves the development of district general hospitals for population areas of around 125,000 during the next ten years.

1968 – The first NHS (and British) heart transplant is made at the National Heart Hospital in London.

1980 – The Black Report investigates the inequality of healthcare. It finds socioeconomic differences in the use of medical services, infant mortality rates and life expectancy.

1981 – The 1981 census shows that 11 babies in every 1,000 died before the age of one. In 1900 this figure was 160. Vaccination programmes, improved sanitation and improved standards of living have vastly increased childhood survival.

1988 – The national breast-screening programme is introduced.

1990 – The NHS and Community Care Act: the introduction of an internal market, whose health authorities manage their own budgets, buying healthcare from other hospitals and providers.

1991 – The first 57 NHS trusts are established, providing health services in the community.

1994 – The NHS Organ Donor Register is established. By 2005 more than 12 million had registered.

1998 – NHS Direct is launched, a nurse-led, 24-hour advice service over the phone.

2000 – NHS walk-in centres are introduced, for the treatment of minor injuries and illnesses without appointment.

2002 – Primary Care Trusts are set up to improve the administration and delivery of healthcare at a local level, liaising with the private sector when contracting out services.

2004 – Patient Choice pilots: everyone referred to hospital treatment is given the choice of at least four hospitals.

2008 – The NHS is one of the largest employers in the world with 1.5 million people. In 2007/08 it had a budget of £90 billion.

Source: Economic and Social Research Council

The GP patient survey 2009/10

Summary

About the surgery or health centre

⇨ The majority of patients find it easy to get into their GP surgery (97%) with four in five (79%) saying it is very easy.

⇨ Almost all patients report their surgery to be clean (98%), with 71% saying it is very clean.

⇨ Nearly nine in ten patients say that other patients can overhear what they say to their surgery's receptionist (86%); however, overall three in five (62%) say they do not mind about this. Only 8% of patients report that they cannot be overheard.

⇨ Overall, patients find their surgery's receptionists to be helpful (93%), with 56% saying they are very helpful.

Getting through on the phone

⇨ Patients were asked about how easy they found it to contact their surgery by phone. Seven in ten patients (68%) say they find it easy to get through to their surgery by phone, with 29% saying it is very easy. While a quarter (25%) say that it is easy to talk to a doctor on the phone, more say that they haven't tried to do this (45%). Similarly, a quarter of patients (24%) say it is easy to speak to a nurse on the phone, but 49% say they have not tried to do this. Over a third of patients (35%) find it easy to get test results on the phone, but again, two in five (40%) have not attempted this.

Seeing a doctor

⇨ Almost two-thirds of patients (64%) have tried to see a doctor fairly quickly in the past six months, and the majority of these (81%) were able to be seen on the same day or within the next two days. The main reason for not being able to be seen, according to patients, was that there were no appointments available (80% mention this).

⇨ Half of patients (50%) have tried to book ahead for an appointment with a doctor in the past six months. The majority of those who tried to book ahead (72%) were able to get an appointment more than two full weekdays in advance. A quarter of patients (25%) were not able to book ahead.

Overall satisfaction

Most patients are satisfied with the care they receive at their surgery (91%), including 56% who are very satisfied. Only 4% are dissatisfied.

When asked how long after their appointment time they normally wait to be seen, only 11% say they are seen at their appointment time

---

⇨ Most patients have seen a doctor at their surgery in the last six months (78%). Of the 22% who have not been seen at their surgery in the last six months, the main reason, perhaps unsurprisingly, is that they have not needed to visit (89% mention this).

Waiting time in the GP surgery or health centre

⇨ When asked how long after their appointment time they normally wait to be seen, only 11% say they are seen at their appointment time. The largest proportion of patients say between five and 15 minutes (49%) and only 6% say they wait more than 30 minutes.

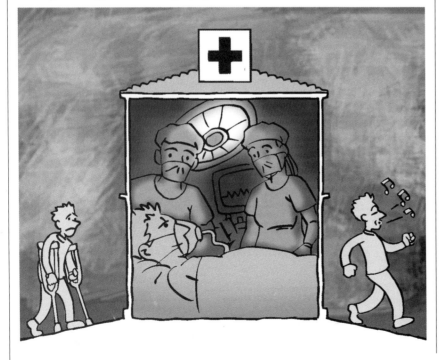

Most patients feel that they do not normally have to wait too long (66%), but 6% say they have to wait far too long.

Seeing the doctor you prefer

⇨ Three in five patients (62%) prefer to see a particular doctor, while 33% say they do not have a preference. Of those who do have a preference, 55% say they always or almost always see this doctor and a further 20% say they see him or her a lot of the time.

Opening hours

⇨ Most patients (81%) are satisfied with the opening hours of their surgery (including 43% who are very satisfied), but 54% would still like their surgery to open at additional times. The clear preference for an additional opening time is on Saturdays, with 54% saying this, compared with 27% who say after 6.30pm. Sundays, at lunchtime and before 8am are least favoured (3%, 6% and 9%, respectively).

Seeing a doctor in the GP surgery or health centre

⇨ Patients were asked a range of questions about the last time they were seen by a doctor at their surgery. The majority of patients are very positive about their experiences with their doctor.

⇨ Most say that their doctor is good at the following: giving enough time (89%), asking about symptoms (88%), listening to them (88%), treating them with care and concern (84%), taking their problems seriously (83%), explaining tests and treatments (78%), and involving them in decisions about their care (73%).

⇨ Importantly, the vast majority of patients (94%) have confidence and trust in the doctor they saw, with 70% saying they definitely have confidence and trust in him or her. Only 4% say they do not.

Seeing a practice nurse in the GP surgery or health centre

⇨ Over half of patients have seen a practice nurse at their surgery in the past six months (54%). Of

those, the majority say it is easy to get an appointment with a nurse (91%), with 53% saying it is very easy.

Most patients (81%) are satisfied with the opening hours of their surgery (including 43% who are very satisfied), but 54% would still like their surgery to open at additional times

---

⇨ The majority of patients are very positive about their experiences with a nurse at their surgery. Most say the nurse was good at the following: giving enough time (84%), treating them with care and concern (80%), listening to them (79%), explaining tests and treatments (74%), asking about symptoms (73%), taking their problems seriously (73%) and involving them in decisions about their care (65%).

Planning your care

⇨ Half of patients (49%) say they have one or more long-standing health problem, disability, or infirmity. Of these, 84% say they have had discussions with a doctor or nurse about how best to deal with their health problem.

⇨ Those who have had discussions about how best to deal with their health problem report different experiences. Nearly nine in ten (88%) felt that the doctor or nurse took notice of their views about dealing with their health problem, and 88% say they were given information on the things they might do to deal with their problem. Similarly, 84% agreed with the doctor or nurse about how best to manage their health problem. However, only 20% say they were given a written document about the discussions they had, and only 12% say that the doctor or nurse ever told them that they had a 'care plan'.

⇨ Overall, the majority of patients with a long-term health problem (88%) think that having discussions with a doctor or nurse has helped improve how they manage their health problem, with 41% saying this has definitely helped.

Out of hours care

⇨ Two-thirds of patients would know how to contact an out-of-hours GP service if they needed to, when their surgery was closed (65%). However, 35% say they would not know how to do this.

⇨ Only 14% of patients have tried to call an out-of-hours GP service when their surgery was closed, either for themselves or for someone else. Of these most patients found it easy to contact the service (79%), with 39% saying it was very easy.

⇨ Half of patients were prescribed or recommended medicines by the out-of-hours service (52%), and of these people 85% found it easy to get hold of these medicines.

⇨ Almost two-thirds (63%) felt that the time it took to receive care from the out-of-hours GP service was about right. However, three in ten felt it took too long (29%).

⇨ Overall, most patients rate the care they received from the out-of-hours service as good (66%), although one in ten rate it as poor (13%).

⇨ The above information is reprinted with kind permission from Ipsos MORI. Please visit www.ipsos-mori.com for more information.

© Ipsos MORI

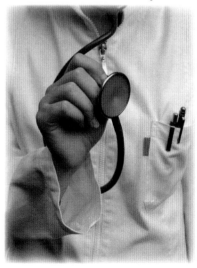

Doctors once again the most trusted profession

Information from the Royal College of Physicians

Doctors have been named the profession most trusted by the general public for the 25th year running,[1] according to the latest Ipsos MORI survey commissioned by the Royal College of Physicians. The annual poll indicates that over nine in ten adults in Britain believe doctors can be trusted to tell the truth, coming ahead of, for example, teachers, professors and judges.

More than 2,000 adults were asked by Ipsos MORI to say whether they generally trusted 16 different types of people to tell the truth or not. More than 90% of the public (92%) said they trusted doctors to tell the truth when the survey was conducted in late 2008. Doctors were closely followed by teachers (87%). The next most trusted were: professors (79%), judges (78%) and clergymen/priests (74%), completing the top five.

At the other end of the scale, only about one in four adults says they trust Government Ministers to tell the truth (24%), and only one in five trusts politicians in general (21%). Journalists move up a non-significant percentage point from 2007, but remain among the lowest ranked, and this year come last with just 19% trusting them to tell the truth.

There was an overall drop in trust across the board in the 2007 study.[2] In a number of cases, the increases in trust seen in 2008 restore the figures to 2006 levels.

Comparison between the 2006 and 2008 figures reveals that the most notable changes are for the ordinary man/woman in the street to tell the truth (a four percentage point increase) – perhaps suggesting greater empowerment of ordinary citizens; trade union officials (+4); the police (+4); judges (+3) and pollsters (-3, but up three points on 2007).

Professor Ian Gilmore, President of the Royal College of Physicians,

said: 'While this remains reassuring for the medical profession, there is no room for complacency. The trust of patients in the modern world has to be earned and retained, and we can do this only by carefully reviewing the changing needs of patients in all aspects of their care. This will include the timely provision of information and the involvement of patients in a true partnership in decisions about their treatment. We are fortunate in having an active patient and carer network integrated into the College to ensure that their views are central to our work.'

Sir Robert Worcester, Founder of Ipsos MORI, said: 'It is a media myth that people are losing trust generally, and specifically that they are losing trust in doctors. In 1983, 82% said they trusted doctors to tell the truth; now this is up ten points, to 92%.

'The stability of these figures across the board is most revealing about the trust people have in the various occupations. Over the past 15 years, on average, the overall level of trust has not varied from 54%, plus or minus three percentage points.

'In the 25 years that MORI has measured the "veracity" of these types of people most have remained stable throughout, only doctors (up ten points), teachers (up eight points), civil servants (up 23 points), trade union officials (up 27 points) and Government Ministers (up eight points) going up by more than five points. The only group down by more than five points is the clergy (down 11).'

Notes

1 Doctors have come first on the list of most trusted professions every year since the MORI poll began in 1983, including one year (1993) when they were joint first with teachers.

2 This was with the exception of judges, for whom trust increased by three percentage points; and Government Ministers for whom the figure remained stable, and at a low level. (Furthermore, the one percentage point fall for journalists from a low level, was not significant.)
12 February 2009

⇨ The above information is reprinted with kind permission from the Royal College of Physicians. Please visit www.rcplondon.ac.uk for more information.

© *Royal College of Physicians*

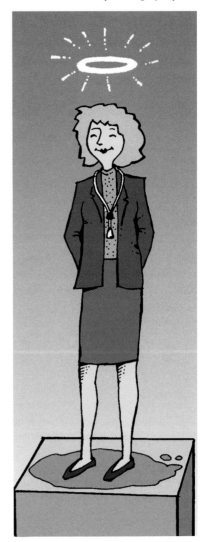

'Evil and Orwellian'

America's right turns its fire on the NHS

The National Health Service has become the butt of increasingly outlandish political attacks in the USA as Republicans and conservative campaigners rail against Britain's 'socialist' system as part of a tussle to defeat Barack Obama's proposals for broader government involvement in healthcare.

Top-ranking Republicans have joined bloggers and well-funded free market organisations in scorning the NHS for its waiting lists and for 'rationing' the availability of expensive treatments.

As myths and half-truths circulate, British diplomats in the USA are treading a delicate line in correcting falsehoods while trying to stay out of a vicious domestic dogfight over the future of American health policy.

Slickly produced television advertisements trumpet the alleged failures of the NHS's 61-year tradition of tax-funded healthcare. To the dismay of British healthcare professionals, US critics have accused the service of putting an 'Orwellian' financial cap on the value on human life, of allowing elderly people to die untreated and, in one case, of driving a despairing dental patient to mend his teeth with superglue.

Having seen his approval ratings drop, Obama is seeking to counter this conservative onslaught by taking his message to the public, with a 'town hall' meeting today at a school in New Hampshire.

Last week, the most senior Republican on the Senate finance committee, Chuck Grassley, took NHS-baiting to a newly emotive level by claiming that his ailing Democratic colleague, Edward Kennedy, would be left to die untreated from a brain tumour in Britain on the grounds that he would be considered too old to deserve treatment.

'I don't know for sure,' said Grassley. 'But I've heard several senators say that Ted Kennedy with a brain tumour, being 77 years old

By Andrew Clark in New York

as opposed to being 37 years old, if he were in England, would not be treated for his disease, because end of life – when you get to be 77, your life is considered less valuable under those systems.'

The degree of misinformation is causing dismay in NHS circles. Andrew Dillon, chief executive of the National Institute for Health and Clinical Excellence (NICE), pointed out that it was utterly false that Kennedy would be left untreated in Britain: 'It is neither true nor is it anything you could extrapolate from anything we've ever recommended to the NHS.'

The National Health Service has become the butt of increasingly outlandish political attacks in the US

Others in the USA have accused Obama of trying to set up 'death panels' to decide who should live and who should die, along the lines of NICE, which determines the cost-effectiveness of NHS drugs.

One right-leaning group, Conservatives for Patients' Rights, lists horror stories about British care on its website. An email widely circulated among US voters, of uncertain origin, claims that anyone over 59 in Britain is ineligible for treatment for heart disease.

The British embassy in Washington is quietly trying to counter inaccuracies. A spokesman said: 'We're keeping a close eye on things and where there's a factually wrong statement, we will take the opportunity to

correct people in private. That said, we don't want to get involved in a domestic debate.'

A $1.2m television advertising campaign bankrolled by the conservative Club for Growth displays images of the union flag and Big Ben while intoning a figure of $22,750. A voiceover says: 'In England, Government health officials have decided that's how much six months of life is worth. If a medical treatment costs more, you're out of luck.'

The number is based on a ratio of £30,000 a year used by NICE in its assessment of whether drugs provide value for money. Dillon said this was one of many variables in determining cost-effectiveness of medicines. He said of his body's portrayal in the USA: 'It's very disappointing and it's not, obviously, the way in which NICE describes itself or the way in which we're perceived in the UK even among those who are disappointed or upset by our decisions.'

On Rupert Murdoch's Fox News channel, the conservative commentator Sean Hannity recently alighted upon the case of Gordon Cook, a security manager from Merseyside, who used superglue to stick a loose crown into his gum because he was unable to find an NHS dentist. The cautionary tale, which was based on a *Daily Mail* report from 2006, prompted Hannity to warn his viewers: 'If the Democrats have their way, get your superglue ready.'

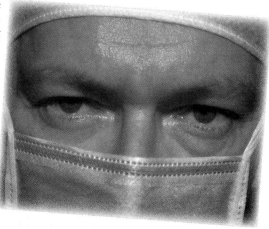

The broader tone of the US healthcare debate has become increasingly bitter. The former vice-presidential candidate Sarah Palin last week described president Obama's proposals as 'evil', while the radio presenter Rush Limbaugh has compared a logo used for the White House's reform plans to a Nazi swastika. Hecklers have disrupted town hall meetings called to discuss the health reform plans.

David Levinthal, a spokesman for the nonpartisan Centre for Responsive Politics, said the sheer scale of the issue, which will affect the entire trajectory of US medical care, was arousing passions: 'It's no surprise you have factions from every political stripe attempting to influence the debate and some of those groups are certainly playing to the deepest fears of Americans. There's been a great deal of documented disinformation propagated throughout the country.' Defenders of Britain's system point out that the UK spends less per head on healthcare but has a higher life expectancy than the USA. The World Health Organization ranks Britain's healthcare as 18th in the world, while the USA is in 37th place. The British Medical Association said a majority of Britain's doctors have consistently supported public provision of healthcare. A spokeswoman said the association's 140,000 members were sceptical about the US approach to medicine: 'Doctors and the public here are appalled that there are so many people on the US who don't have proper access to healthcare. It's something we would find very, very shocking.'
11 August 2009

© *Guardian Newspapers Ltd*

Why we love the NHS

A UNISON factsheet specially prepared for sister unions in the USA

The UK's National Health Service provides a comprehensive range of services that is free at the point of need and accessible to all. It provides peace of mind to millions, regardless of their income or employment circumstances.

The NHS has come under attack from right-wing critics of President Obama's health plans. Some of these claims, such as those that patients over a certain age cannot receive treatment for brain tumours or heart bypasses, are simply untrue – there are no such bans and nor have there ever been.

Various rogue British commentators, such as Daniel Hannan and Karol Sikora, are trying to portray the NHS as dysfunctional or describing it as a '60-year mistake'. However, as the facts and figures below demonstrate, nothing could be further from the truth.

Is the NHS an efficient system?

⇨ OECD figures show that UK total health expenditure as a percentage of GDP (8.4%) is actually below the OECD average and a long way below that of the USA, which has easily the most expensive system at 16%, nearly double UK spending.

⇨ The UK spend per head of population is $2,992 as opposed to $7,290 in the USA.

⇨ The UK NHS is largely free of the huge transaction costs associated with revenue collection and marketing that blight other systems, such as the USA. As a result, the cost of administration in the UK is estimated at around 12% compared to more than 30% in the USA.

⇨ The UK spends 3% of its budget on management costs, as opposed to 17% in the USA.

⇨ The NHS has not been complacent or uncritically carried on as normal; a major review at the start of this decade evaluated different healthcare funding options and concluded that the current method of NHS funding through general taxation was both the fairest and most efficient one.

⇨ Productivity in the NHS has been rising alongside recent extra funding, for example by 0.7% in 2006 and by 1.2% in 2007.

What are the waiting times for treatment on the NHS?

⇨ From January 2009, no one in England waits more than 18 weeks from the time they are referred to the start of their treatment. Most importantly, the average wait for treatment is much shorter, at just eight weeks. And median waiting times are just over two weeks for outpatients and four weeks for inpatients.

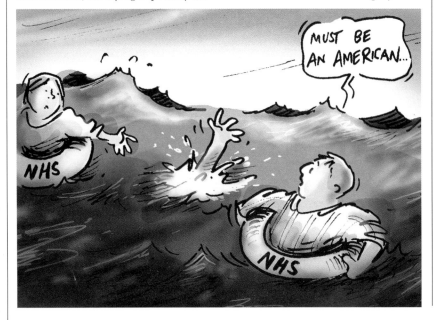

- For cancer patients, 99.7% of patients are seen within two weeks from urgent GP referral to outpatient appointment. For breast cancer, 99.8% of patients are treated within one month from diagnosis to treatment.
- Virtually all patients are treated within four hours at Accident & Emergency units in hospitals.

How is the NHS performing?

- Claims that clinical outcomes in the NHS are lagging behind other countries, particularly the USA, are wide of the mark.
- For example, the UK outperforms the USA where mortality rates from lung cancers are concerned.
- Likewise, UK mortality rates from heart disease and stroke are considerably better than the USA.
- And in terms of in-hospital recovery from stroke, the UK is ranked second only to Japan amongst the OECD countries.

How does the UK system compare to others?

- In comparison with the healthcare systems of five other comparable countries (Australia, Canada, Germany, New Zealand and the USA) the NHS was found to be the most impressive overall by the New York-based Commonwealth Fund in 2007 (the USA came last). Specifically the NHS was rated as the best system in terms of quality of care, co-ordination of care, and equity, but also, crucially, in terms of the efficiency of care.
- The last time the World Health Organization produced a ranking of the world's health systems, the UK was ranked considerably higher than the USA.
- Life expectancy at birth is greater in the UK than in the USA and the infant mortality rate is lower in the UK than in the USA.

What is NICE?

- Far from being a 'death panel', the National Institute for healthcare and Clinical Excellence (NICE) is a world-renowned body that evaluates the effectiveness of drugs for use in the UK health system.

- NICE does not put a limit on the amount the NHS can spend on an individual patient.
- Its evaluation process involves top medical experts working alongside members of the public and many other health systems in the world are now looking to duplicate its approach to drug evaluation.

NICE does not put a limit on the amount the NHS can spend on an individual patient

---

- NICE rejects only a tiny percentage of all the drugs it assesses for use on the NHS (around 5%) and since 1999 has recommended over 90% of the cancer drugs it has been asked to look at.

What do patients think of their NHS?

- The NHS remains a defining feature of life in the UK, consistently rated as more popular than the Royal Family or Parliament.
- The NHS regulator's latest patient survey recorded 92% of patients saying their care was 'good', 'very good' or 'excellent'.
- According to the 2009 British Social Attitudes report, satisfaction with the NHS is at its highest level for 25 years. And those with personal experience of the NHS rate it highest of all.

What do people say about the NHS?

- Professor Stephen Hawking: 'I wouldn't be here today if it were not for the NHS. I have received a large amount of high-quality treatment without which I would not have survived.'
- Explorer Sir Ranulph Fiennes: 'I love the NHS because they saved me from certain death following a massive heart attack. Also, when my wife of 36 years was terminally ill with cancer the NHS looked after her diligently and with expertise and patience.'
- Prime Minister Gordon Brown: 'The NHS makes the difference

between pain and comfort, life and death.'
- UNISON General Secretary Dave Prentis: 'Regardless of your income, the NHS provides peace of mind even at the most uncertain economic times, like those we're experiencing now. In the US, losing your job means losing your health insurance.'

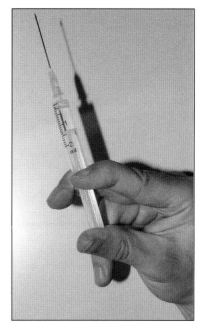

About UNISON

UNISON is a powerful voice for working people in the UK. We have over 1.3 million members working in public services, the community and voluntary sector and for private companies. UNISON is the UK's largest healthcare trade union – representing 400,000 nurses, student nurses, midwives, health visitors, healthcare assistants, paramedics, cleaners, porters, catering staff, medical secretaries, clerical and admin staff and scientific and technical staff.

UNISON campaigns for quality public services as the foundation of a strong economy and a fair society. Add your voice to ours at www.unison.org.uk/million
August 2009

- The above information is reprinted with kind permission from UNISON, the public service union. Please visit www.unison.org.uk for more information, or to view references for this article.

© UNISON

What is NICE and how does it work?

This article explains the work of the National Institute for Health and Clinical Excellence (NICE)

What NICE is

NICE stands for the National Institute for Health and Clinical Excellence. It is an independent organisation, and was set up by the Government in 1999. NICE decides which drugs and treatments are available on the NHS in England and Wales. Scotland and Northern Ireland have separate organisations to make decisions.

The Government developed NICE to get rid of 'the postcode lottery' – where some drugs and treatments were available in some parts of the country, but not in others. NICE aims to give independent advice about which treatments should be available on the NHS in England and Wales, and to make sure that people have the same access to treatment and care wherever they live.

What NICE does

NICE's main functions are:
⇨ To assess new drugs and treatments as they become available;
⇨ To provide guidelines on how a particular condition should be treated.

NICE considers whether a treatment:
⇨ Benefits patients;
⇨ Will help the NHS meet its targets, for example by improving cancer survival rates;
⇨ Is value for money, or cost effective.

Once NICE issues its guidance, NHS trusts and primary care organisations must find the money to make those drugs or treatments available. NICE doesn't give any extra money, or advise on how to find the money.

When making decisions, NICE asks for expert advice from:
⇨ Medical and other health professionals;
⇨ Patients and patient organisations;
⇨ Drug companies.

How NICE works

The Department of Health (DOH) for England and the National Assembly for Wales (NAW) decide which topics NICE will look at. Anyone can suggest a topic for NICE. You just need to fill out a form on the NICE website (it's in the 'suggest a topic' section). You can complete the form online, or print and post it.

Making a suggestion doesn't mean that NICE will look at it. The DOH has guidelines to help them decide which topics to choose.

NICE divides its guidance into three main areas:

⇨ Health technology – specific medicines, treatments and procedures;
⇨ Clinical practice – how doctors and nurses should treat diseases and conditions;
⇨ Public health – preventing illness and health promotion.

How NICE makes a decision

It can take 18 months or more for NICE to decide if a drug or treatment should be available. NICE makes its decisions based on:
⇨ Evidence – NICE reviews each treatment or new technique;
⇨ Cost effectiveness – including the quality-of-life-adjusted-year (QALY);
⇨ Contributions from patient organisations, health professionals, experts, and other interested parties.

A QALY is a tool that takes into account how a treatment affects:
⇨ Quantity of life;
⇨ Quality of life.

'Quantity of life' means how long someone lives for. 'Quality of life' is more about how the treatment affects you. It includes:
⇨ How well you are;
⇨ Whether you can work;
⇨ Whether you can care for yourself.

Some NICE decisions have been in the news lately. NICE now has a 'fast track' procedure, which aims to make reviews of new treatments and medical techniques available more quickly. All drugs need a licence before doctors can prescribe them on the NHS. With the fast track procedure, NICE can look at some drugs while they are still in the licensing stage, rather than waiting until after they are licensed. This means that NICE can make a decision very quickly after the drug has been licensed. You can find out more about how drugs are licensed in our cancer treatment questions.

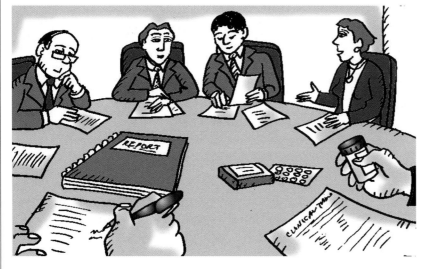

The NHS should use NICE guidance as soon as it is published. Your doctors will still use their knowledge and skills to decide the best treatment for you.

Your local area NHS should find the money to fund technology guidance, usually within three months of NICE issuing guidance.

It can take 18 months or more for NICE to decide if a drug or treatment should be available

When NICE issues clinical practice guidance, the NHS and health professionals will need to decide if they are already meeting the requirements in the guidance, or need to change the treatment and care that they provide.

Scotland and Northern Ireland

There is a slightly different process in Scotland and Northern Ireland.

Scotland

In Scotland the following organisations perform a similar function to NICE:

⇨ The NHS Quality Improvement for Scotland carries out technology appraisals;

⇨ The Scottish Intercollegiate Guidelines Network (SIGN) provides clinical guidelines;

⇨ The Scottish Medicines Consortium (SMC) gives immediate advice on new medicines when they become available.

NHS Quality Improvement for Scotland

This organisation provides Health Technology Appraisals for Scotland. Like NICE, they gather evidence and contributions from patient organisations and experts to make a decision about a particular topic.

Scottish Intercollegiate Guidelines Network (SIGN)

The members of this network include patients and their carers, health professionals and other professionals involved in caring for people, such as social workers and managers. SIGN aims to improve the quality of health

care for people in Scotland by making sure everyone gets the same, good standard of care.

Northern Ireland

The Department of Health, Social Services and Public Safety (HPSS) in Northern Ireland agreed in July 2006 to link to NICE. This means that they will look at any guidance issued by NICE and decide if it is relevant for Northern Ireland.

If NICE's guidance isn't relevant, or if the HPSS decide it's only partly relevant, they will advise on any changes that need to be made. The HPSS are likely to approve most NICE guidance. The Department usually makes a decision shortly after NICE has made their decision.

Appeals

Patient organisations can comment on a piece of guidance while NICE are still developing it. There is also an appeals process and those with an interest can appeal against a decision. NICE call these interested parties 'stakeholders'.

Stakeholders include:

⇨ Patient organisations;

⇨ Health professionals;

⇨ Companies that make any of the treatments for that particular condition;

⇨ Health service providers;

⇨ Statutory organisations, such as the DOH and NAW.

You have to be a registered stakeholder to be able to appeal to NICE.

Getting drugs before a NICE decision

Your doctor can prescribe a drug for you while NICE are looking at it – if your local NHS trust agrees that they can. Once NICE makes a decision, it replaces any decision made locally.

NICE don't licence drugs or new devices. The Medicines and Healthcare products Regulatory Agency (MHRA) does this. Your local NHS decides whether a drug or device should be prescribed. NICE looks at them:

⇨ If there is uncertainty about whether they should be prescribed; and

⇨ To ensure you have access to

treatment and care wherever you live.

What to do if you can't get a drug

First, it's always best to talk to your specialist about your treatment. There may be good reasons why you aren't having a particular treatment.

If it's a drug that NICE have approved, read the guidance to check exactly who it says should have the drug or treatment. It may be that the guidance says that you should have the drug only after another treatment has not worked, or is no longer working. NICE writes versions of their decisions for the public, which can be easier to read. You can find them on the NICE website.

Points to consider include:

⇨ Is this the best treatment for your cancer at this particular time?

⇨ Are there any reasons why you shouldn't have the treatment, for example side effects?

If it is a drug that NICE have not approved, you need to talk to your specialist about it. If your doctor agrees that the treatment would help to control your cancer, you can apply to your Primary Care Trust (PCT) for 'exceptional funding'. The PCT has to keep some money aside for these claims. It will probably take quite a bit of time and effort, but people do sometimes succeed in getting treatments funded this way. You may also find it helpful to contact a patient organisation, as they can often offer help and support. They may know of others who have gone down this route.

After doing all this, if you still believe you aren't getting the right treatment, contact the Patient Advice and Liaison Service (PALS). There will be one within your local hospital. They can help you resolve the problem. If it still isn't sorted out, contact the Care Quality Commission. They can investigate the complaint.

⇨ Taken from CancerHelp UK, the patient information website of Cancer Research UK: www.cancerhelp.org. uk. Reprinted with permission of Cancer Research UK.

© Cancer Research UK

Should NHS offer incentives to improve health?

A new research centre that will study the ethics, economics and psychology behind the use of incentives in healthcare has opened

Giving people financial incentives to change their behaviour or adhere to medication regimens is becoming a more frequent approach adopted by healthcare providers around the world, often attracting controversy.

For example, some Primary Care Trusts (PCTs) in the UK offer vouchers to pregnant women who manage to give up smoking for a set period of time; and some patients receive around £10 each time they receive prescribed medication for psychotic disorders.

The Centre for the Study of Incentives in Healthcare (CSI Health) is a collaboration between King's College London, the London School of Economics and Political Science (LSE), and Queen Mary, University of London (QMUL). It is funded by an £800,000 Strategic Award in Biomedical Ethics from the Wellcome Trust.

Research at CSI Health will address the use of incentives to change people's behaviour from the perspectives of three main disciplines – philosophy, psychology and economics – with the aim of evaluating whether financial incentives are an effective and acceptable means by which to improve population health.

The Director of the new Centre is Theresa Marteau, Professor of Health Psychology at King's College London. 'Financial incentives provide immediate rewards for behaviours that may only otherwise reap rewards in the future,' says Professor Marteau. 'These include stopping smoking or eating fruit, for example.

'They also capitalise on "present bias" – a tendency most of us have to pursue small immediate rewards rather than more distant ones, even those that are far more highly valued. The theory is that by establishing

wellcometrust

new behaviours using the power of rewards, these new behaviours will become habitual.'

Incentives have proved effective, particularly in developing countries where they have been used to encourage one-off behaviours like clinic attendance or vaccinations. Changing habitual behaviours has proved more difficult.

Giving people financial incentives to change their behaviour or adhere to medication regimens is becoming a more frequent approach adopted by healthcare providers

---

Adam Oliver, health economist at LSE and co-director of CSI Health, says: 'The failure of incentives to change behaviour in the long term could be because the schemes have not drawn upon psychological or behavioural economic theory.

'There are objections to the use of incentives,' says Richard Ashcroft, Professor of Biomedical Ethics at QMUL and co-director of CSI Health. 'These objections seem to derive from a view that incentives are a form of bribery or coercion, or that it is unfair to "reward" people

who have previously chosen to engage in less healthy behaviour. So at CSI Health we will go beyond asking simply whether incentives work. We will examine whether incentives produce sustained health benefits, and what impact they have beyond the individual patient.'

Clare Matterson, Director of Medicine, Society and History at the Wellcome Trust, says: 'Research into ethical issues surrounding medical science and healthcare is essential if people are going to be able to make informed decisions about their own behaviour and its impact on their health.

'By funding the Centre for the Study of Incentives in Health, we expect Professor Marteau and her colleagues to really move research on in this field over the next five years, extending international collaborations and developing new ways of multidisciplinary working in what is a complicated and controversial area of health policy.'
30 April 2009

⇨ The above information is reprinted with kind permission from the Wellcome Trust. Visit www.wellcome. ac.uk for more information.
© *Wellcome Trust*

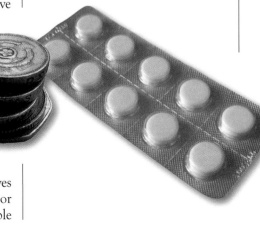

Has the NHS been successful?

Information from the Office of Health Economics

It is difficult to be objective about the NHS. Most people seem to feel passionately about it. Many believe as Bevan did that 'no society can legitimately call itself civilised if a sick person is denied medical aid because of lack of means'. In their view the NHS makes us a civilised society and they cannot speak too highly of the quality of the care and the dedication of the doctors and nurses.

It is difficult to be objective about the NHS. Most people seem to feel passionately about it

---

Others take the view expressed by Jonathan Miller writing in the *Sunday Times*:

'It is an enduring eccentricity of the British that we regard our National Health Service as the envy of the world, despite the evidence staring us in the face of slum hospitals staffed by surly trade unionists (the doctors surliest of all) and run by vast legions of bureaucrats accountable to nobody, least of all the customers.'

Positive achievements

The positive achievements of the NHS could be summarised as follows.

1 The NHS is cheap by international standards. For example, the UK spent 7.1% of Gross Domestic Product (GDP) on healthcare in 2000, most of this on the NHS, while the average for the rest of the European Union (EU) in 1998 (latest data available) was 9.2%.

2 The level of health in the UK is similar to that in other developed countries. For example, the life expectancy of a male in the UK born between 1990 and 1995 was 73.7 years whereas the average for the EU was 73.2 years. The corresponding figures for females are 79.0 years in the UK as against 79.6 in the rest of the EU.

3 The NHS has avoided many of the problems of insurance-based health care systems:

⇨ Doctors are either salaried or under contract to the NHS. They are not normally paid a fee for service for NHS work. This has avoided over-supply problems.

⇨ Doctors decide who needs treatment. In particular, GPs act as both a guide (to the appropriate specialist) and as a filter. This both helps overcome the problems of consumer ignorance and provides a means of controlling the level of demand.

⇨ Since healthcare is funded by taxation and is free at the point of use, there are no gaps in the system and no stigma attached to receiving care.

⇨ The budget for the NHS is determined centrally. The Secretary of State for Health negotiates with the Treasury and the decision is then ratified in Cabinet and voted on in Parliament. This budget determines the quantity of resources available for the NHS and thus provides a way of explicitly setting the maximum amount of healthcare that can be available to NHS patients as a whole.

4 The NHS has continued to be popular. Klein has commented that 'the NHS seems to be a remarkably successful instrument for making the rationing of scarce resources socially and politically acceptable'.

Barr argues that the NHS has been successful because it has resolved many of the problems which face healthcare systems – 'an institution which arose

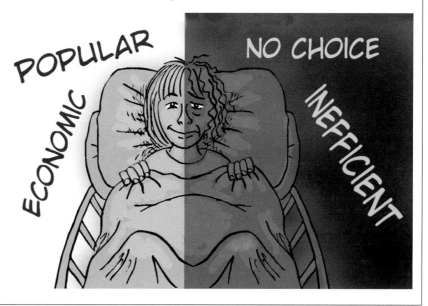

historically largely for equity reasons works because it goes with the grain of efficiency considerations'.

Serious problems

What about the criticisms of the NHS? Many people believe that the NHS suffers from serious problems.

1 The critics argue that insufficient resources have been devoted to healthcare so that there is less care than consumers would like. This is a consequence of funding the service from taxation – there is no mechanism whereby consumers can signal their willingness to pay more. According to this view the fact that the UK spends less of its GDP on healthcare than other developed countries reflects a weakness of the NHS rather than evidence of its efficiency. This also explains why the NHS appears to be in continual financial crisis – waiting lists, closed wards and an inability to treat particular patients or particular conditions all reflect a failure to devote sufficient resources to healthcare.

2 The system is not sensitive to consumer preferences. Doctors have considerable independence or clinical autonomy. They make decisions about patients' treatment with little reference to either the patients or the managerial structure of the NHS. This has resulted in a system which is unwieldy and difficult to control and not responsive to consumer demand.

3 The NHS is not as efficient as it could be. Some hospitals need to be closed and the resources transferred into community healthcare. But opponents, including some doctors, have successfully delayed, and in some cases prevented, such changes from occurring. They argue that the closure of any hospital is a loss of NHS services regardless of how the resources made available may be used to provide other, more valuable, kinds of healthcare.

⇨ The above information is reprinted with kind permission from the Office of Health Economics. Please visit their website at www.ohe.org for more information.

© OHE 2009 www.ohe.org

Patients not numbers, people not statistics

Patients Association releases shocking accounts of NHS hospital care

PA publishes 'Patients not Numbers, People not statistics' – 16 first-hand accounts of patient care in hospital.

The Patients Association has campaigned for many years to improve the quality of care provided by the NHS and throughout that time our efforts have been fuelled by the accounts we receive on a daily basis from patients and their relatives through our helpline.

As a consistent pattern of shocking standards of care has emerged we have decided to publish a number of these accounts to highlight the unacceptable experiences facing patients up and down the country on a regular basis. The Patients Association calls on Government

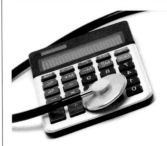

and the Care Quality Commission to conduct an urgent review of the standards of basic care being received by patients in hospital and demands stricter supervision and regulation of hospital care.

Director of the Patients Association Katherine Murphy said: 'Whilst mid-Staffordshire may have been an anomaly in terms of scale, the PA knew the kinds of appalling treatment given there could be found across the NHS. This report removes any doubt and makes this clear to all. Two of the accounts come from Stafford, and they sadly fail to stand out from the others.

'These accounts tell the story of the two per cent of patients that consistently rate their care as poor. If this was extrapolated to the whole of the NHS from 2002 to 2008 it would equate to over one million patients. Very often these are the most vulnerable elderly and terminally ill

patients – it's a sad indictment of the care they receive.

'These accounts reveal patients being denied basic dignity in their care – often left in soiled bedclothes, being given inadequate food and drink, having repeated falls, suffering from late diagnosis, cancelled operations, bungled referrals and misplaced notes. There are also worrying instances of cruel and callous attitudes from staff towards vulnerable and sometimes terminally ill patients.

'These accounts tell the story of the two per cent of patients that consistently rate their care as poor'

'We hope this report is a wake-up call for the Department of Health and the Care Quality Commission – we've made a number of recommendations to try and prevent these kinds of things happening to other patients. We hope this report also encourages other people to get in touch with us and tell their stories – we plan to continue publishing accounts until we can be confident that every patient is secured dignity in their care. The people that have come forward for this report are incredibly brave and had one thing in common – they want it stopped.'

President of the Patients Association Claire Rayner said: 'For far too long now, the Patients Association has been receiving calls on our helpline from people wanting to talk about the dreadful, neglectful, demeaning, painful and sometimes downright cruel treatment their elderly relatives had experienced at the hands of NHS nurses.

'I am sickened by what has happened to some part of my profession of which I was so proud. These bad, cruel nurses may be – probably are – a tiny proportion of the nursing work force, but even if they are only one or two per cent of the whole they should be identified and struck off the Register.

'One Hospital Trust has raised the spectre of legal action if we publish this material, others have been unhelpful, not answering relatives' letters and not investigating their complaints. The personal accounts given here are just a few of those brought to us.'

Extracts from the accounts

Account 1: Leslie Kirk

'Toilets were not cleaned properly with faeces clearly left from several previous uses. My sister often had to clean them herself before she'd let my father use them.'

'At no time during my father's stay on the ward did we feel there was anyone who cared for patients enough and who took responsibility for ensuring they got the attention they needed.'

Account 2: Pamela Goddard

'Upsettingly for my brother who visited her frequently, she was often found in her own faeces and urine when he arrived. He would need to prompt staff to come and wash and change her.'

Account 3: Florence Weston

'She was also told that, because of being unable to use the toilet facilities through being immobile, she should wet the bed. This was highly embarrassing for her. Even worse, on one occasion, a night nurse told her off for doing this severely enough to reduce her to tears and cause her to ask me if she could go home.'

Account 4: Oenone Hewlett

'When she arrived at Wexham Accident and Emergency following her stay at St Marks, the doctor thought she must have been at home alone and neglecting herself. We had to explain she had been in hospital. He couldn't understand how she could've become so dehydrated.'

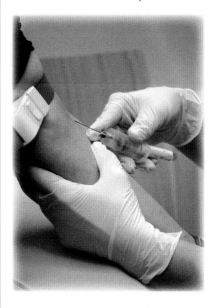

Account 5: Bella Bailey

'Confused patients often wandered around semi naked and some staff passed them by in the corridor without a care. Night time and weekends were the worst. Night time was often the most busiest and noisiest. Staff squealed and giggled whilst patients tried to grab a bit of sleep in between their discomforts.'

Account 6: Thomas Milner

'The nurse also failed to provide incontinence pads as had been done during the evening and night before. He was bleeding rectally and he ended up laying in urine and blood. He also wet the floor and my elderly mother wiped this up while the nurse and assistant nurse watched on and did nothing to help. They did not even bring a mop and bucket afterwards to disinfect the floor.'

Account 7: Anne McNeill

'I remember on one occasion I visited her and found her sitting in a chair with her own vomit all over her clothes. It was dried so it seemed as if it must have been left there for some time. There was also dried vomit in a bowl next to her. I looked up and down the ward and couldn't find a nurse anywhere.'

'Confused patients often wandered around semi naked and some staff passed them by in the corridor without a care'

Account 8: Thomas George Dalziel

'When we were taken to his bed we were not prepared for the horrific sight of seeing him, eyes wide open with a resuscitation tube down his throat. This image has traumatised not only us but also my sister and brother-in-law for the rest of our lives!'

Account 9: Jayne Knowles Smith

'I used to pride myself on being a nurse and hopefully I was caring and thoughtful. I have had the misfortune of seeing nursing from another angle as a patient. It's a scary world out in the wards. I'm not sure if it's the training that's lacking, the basic skills or just understaffing.'

Account 10: Colin Richard Purkiss Smith

'That evening my husband wanted to go to the toilet. I needed help from staff to take him and so I asked staff for help. Over an hour later still no one had come and my husband had an accident in the bed. I went outside of the room to the nursing station to get one of the staff to get clean sheets for the bed and when I looked, I noticed that one of the staff on duty was surfing the Internet.'

Account 11: John David Drake

'I then went to the hospital and when we arrived at the ward, we were both shocked to see the state that my husband was in. My husband appeared very dehydrated and even more confused. My husband had not been washed and neither was there water on my husband's locker. I washed my husband myself and gave him a lot of water to drink. It took some time as it was hard for him to swallow but with some patience and care he was able to drink plenty of water to quench his thirst.'

Account 12: Professor Leslie C Vaughan

'I find it unacceptable that a man at this point so obviously close to the end of his life should be left alone behind a curtain on a busy ward. The staff had phoned us and knew we were coming so that they surely could have spared a sympathetic nurse to sit with him until we arrived.'

Account 13: Margaret Bristo

'Often you would stand right in front of them (the nurses' station) but staff would keep their heads down and avoid eye contact with you. All my brothers and sisters felt the same. One even asked "am I invisible?" after being ignored time and time again.'

Account 14: Alice Fowler

'I witnessed patients struggling to open plastic packages of sandwiches and/ or fruit juice. Sometimes if patients weren't awake during meal times their food was left uncovered without any attempt to wake them or encourage them to eat. The food would then be taken away untouched.'

Account 15: Barbara McVernon

'A few mornings after mum's admission, I arrived to discover a patient with dementia in her room, going through her belongings. When the old lady refused to leave and became aggressive, I rang the nurses' bell but no one responded. I was reduced to shouting down the corridor. Eventually a non-uniformed woman came and led her away.'

Account 16: Patient A

'The toilet was disgusting. It was soiled and had a soiled toilet brush. The public toilets downstairs were bad enough, often dirty and blocked. It's horrifying to see this in a hospital let alone on a ward. There are countries poorer than us yet their hospitals are clean and immaculate.'

August 2009

⇨ Information from the Patients Association. Please visit www.patients-association.org.uk for more.

© *Patients Association*

Common hospital superbugs

An influential group of MPs has warned that the Government has taken its 'eye off the ball' on hospital superbugs. What are these infections? And what can they do to you? By Kate Devlin, Medical Correspondent

MRSA

⇨ Stands for Methicillin-resistant Staphylococcus aureus.
⇨ A common bacteria found on the surface of the skin, it is resistant to a range of antibiotics.
⇨ The bacteria can get into the body through breaks in the skin.
⇨ If it enters the bloodstream it can cause serious infections, such as blood poisoning, and even death.

C. difficile

⇨ Belongs to the same family of bacteria which cause tetanus.
⇨ Usually lives in the large intestine and is found in low numbers in around five per cent of all adults.
⇨ Causes diarrhoea and if not treated properly can even cause death.

MSSA

⇨ Meticillin-susceptible Staphylococcus aureus.
⇨ Similar to MRSA, it can prove equally as deadly.
⇨ Leslie Ash, the actress, contracted MSSA after a stay in hospital in 2004.

E-coli

⇨ A common bacteria, of which many types are harmless.
⇨ However, more serious strains can cause dangerous food poisoning in humans.
⇨ The infection can also prove fatal.

Klebsiella

⇨ Another common bacteria, it can cause a range of illnesses including pneumonia and urinary tract infections.
⇨ A Klebsiella infection can also be deadly.
⇨ Like E-coli there are signs that the bugs are becoming resistant to some commonly used antibiotics.

10 November 2009

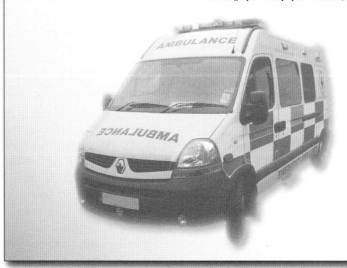

Fall in deaths linked to C. difficile and MRSA

Information from the Office for National Statistics

The number of death certificates in England and Wales mentioning Clostridium difficile or MRSA as a contributory factor fell sharply between 2007 and 2008.

New figures published today by the Office for National Statistics show that death certificates mentioning C. difficile fell by 29 per cent between 2007 and 2008, to 5,931 mentions. This is the first year that mentions have fallen since records began in 1999.

The number of death certificates mentioning meticillin-resistant Staphylococcus aureas, or MRSA, fell by 23 per cent to 1,230. This is the second consecutive year in which mentions have fallen.

Age-standardised death rates for men and women show that deaths involving C. difficile fell by 27 per cent for men and 30 per cent for women between 2007 and 2008.

For MRSA, age-standardised death rates show a decline of 31 per cent and 13 per cent for men and women respectively.

Death rates for both C. difficile and MRSA were higher among the older age groups. For C. difficile, in the 85 and over group, there were 2,331 and 2,303 deaths per million population for men and women, respectively. The corresponding figures for MRSA were 659 and 326 deaths per million population for men and women, respectively.

Between 2004 and 2008, C. difficile was involved in 1 per 1,000 deaths in England and Wales. MRSA was involved in 3 per 1,000 deaths.
19 August 2009

⇨ The above information is reprinted with kind permission from the Office for National Statistics. Please visit www.statistics.gov.uk for more information.
© Crown copyright

England is 'poor relation' of NHS devolution

By David Batty and agencies

The NHS in England has become the poor relation of the service in other parts of the UK, a patients' group said today.

The Patients Association said devolution had led to a widening gap between NHS provision in England and the rest of the UK, with patients in Scotland, Wales and Northern Ireland getting a better deal.

Michael Summers, vice-chairman of the association, said patients in Scotland enjoyed free personal care for the elderly, while those in Wales enjoyed free prescriptions. In contrast, patients in England were means tested for personal care and had to pay for prescriptions.

Summers told BBC Radio 4's *Today* programme: 'I think we should follow best practice. The best practice is that which they have discovered in Scotland, Wales and Northern Ireland.

'They have all said that people should have free prescriptions and that we should look after our elderly people. England, for some reason, seems to have been the poor relation.'

His comments came after the head of the NHS Confederation said there were now four different health services operating in the UK, and that the differences between them were likely to increase.

Dr Gill Morgan, the organisation's chief executive, told the BBC News website: 'We basically have four different systems, albeit with the same set of values.

'This period (since devolution) has been unique in the history of the NHS as it was essentially the same across the UK before devolution. We have had a complete split in philosophy.'

She said England had concentrated on cutting waiting times and offering patients more choice; Scotland had introduced free personal care; Wales had introduced free prescriptions; and Northern Ireland had fully integrated health and social care.

Dr Morgan said it was too early to say which system was more successful as each had its advantages but she said the differences were expected to become even greater.
2 January 2008
© Guardian Newspapers Limited 2010

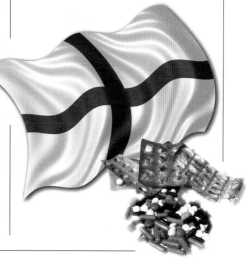

Devolved healthcare

Some UK countries spending more on the NHS but delivering less, finds major new Nuffield Trust report

A unique analysis published today of the performance of the NHS across the four countries of the UK before and after devolution has found striking differences in performance, with some countries spending more on health care and employing greater numbers of health staff but performing worse when it comes to a range of indicators, such as waiting times and crude productivity of staff.

The report by the independent health charity The Nuffield Trust examines the performance of the health services in England, Scotland, Wales and Northern Ireland across three time points – 1996/97, 2002/03 and 2006/07. It also examines the performance of the ten English regions and compares them with the NHS in England as a whole and the NHS in each of the devolved countries in 2006/07. This is the first time such an analysis has been conducted. Performance was tracked against a number of key indicators, including expenditure, staffing levels, activity (outpatient appointments, inpatient admissions and day cases), crude productivity of staff and waiting times.

The main findings are:

⇨ Historically Scotland, Wales and Northern Ireland have had higher levels of funding per capita for NHS care than England. However, the research suggests the NHS in England spends less and has fewer doctors, nurses and managers per head of population than the health services in the devolved countries, but that it is making better use of the resources it has in terms of delivering higher levels of activity, crude productivity of its staff and lower waiting times.

⇨ Scotland has the highest levels of poor health, the highest rates of expenditure, the highest rates of hospital doctors, GPs and nurses per capita, and yet it has the lowest rates of crude productivity of its staff and the lowest rates of

inpatient admissions per head of population in 2006/07.

⇨ In 2006, Wales had the lowest rate of day cases but the highest rate of outpatient attendances, while Northern Ireland had the lowest rate of outpatient attendances but the highest rate of inpatient admissions and day cases.

⇨ The performance of Wales and Northern Ireland in key measures of waiting has been poor compared with England (Scotland's waiting times could not be compared with those of England, Wales and Northern Ireland at the three time points because they were measured in a different way). By 2006, virtually no patients in England waited more than three months for an outpatient appointment, whereas in Wales and Northern Ireland 44 per cent and 61 per cent of patients did. By 2006, virtually all patients in England who needed inpatient or day case treatment were seen within six months, while in Wales and Northern Ireland 79 per cent and 84 per cent of patients waited longer than this.

Dr Jennifer Dixon, director of The Nuffield Trust, said: 'A key question for the NHS in all four countries, especially in the current economic climate, must be whether or not value for money is being obtained. While this research suggests that efficiencies can be made in health services throughout the UK, the marked differences in crude productivity of staff in the three devolved nations relative to England raise challenging questions.

'Some of the differences and trends may be because of the historical differences in funding levels, which are not directly related to policies implemented after devolution. But some will reflect the different policies pursued by each of the four nations since 1999, in particular the greater pressure put on NHS

bodies in England to improve performance in a few key areas such as waiting and efficiency, via targets, strong performance management, public reporting of performance by regulators, and financial incentives.

'We believe the research raises important questions about the efficiency of care across the devolved nations. There is a lack of comparable data that allow differences in performance across the UK to be analysed in depth in future. Without such comparable data, UK taxpayers and HM Treasury cannot know whether they are securing value for money for their health services.'

The report found that the differences in performance on waiting times and staff productivity are more pronounced when the devolved nations are compared with regions of England that are similar on a range of health and socio-economic indicators. Putting London to one side, which distorts the national averages of staff productivity for England,* the devolved nations are still outliers on waiting times and staff productivity relative to English regions that are most similar to them on a range of health and socio-economic indicators.

For example, the north-east of England provides a good benchmark for comparisons with Scotland. In 2006 for a population of 100,000, expenditure in Scotland would have been about £180 million, compared to £170 million for the north-east region. Yet Scotland's six per cent of additional funding resulted in 14 per cent more hospital doctors (205 to 180) and GPs (81 to 71), nearly 50 per cent more nurses (1,100 to 740), and nearly 75 per cent more managers and support staff (730 to 420). Despite its lower level of expenditure and staffing, the north-east region compared with Scotland delivered 18 per cent more outpatient attendances (105,000 to 89,300), almost 40 per cent more day cases

(10,500 to 7,600) and more than 50 per cent more inpatient admissions (20,700 to 13,500). Consequently, the staff in the north-east had far higher levels of crude productivity than in Scotland.

The report looks only at statistics that can be measured in the same way in the English regions and the devolved countries at three selected time points. It is possible that the comparative statistics that are available fail to capture some important dimensions of performance. The report recommends that other dimensions, such as staff and patient experience and health outcomes, should therefore be the subject of further research. However, it also concludes that previously published studies do not point to consistent higher levels of quality of care in the devolved nations that might partly offset the lower crude productivity levels of staff relative to England.

Notes

1 *Funding and Performance of Healthcare Systems in the Four Countries of the UK Before and After Devolution* was written by Sheelah Connolly, Research Fellow, Queen's University Belfast; Professor Nicholas Mays, Professor of Health Policy, London School of Hygiene and Tropical Medicine; and Professor Gwyn Bevan, Professor of Management Science, London School of Economics & Political Science. Full biographies and a full copy of the report are available on request. The report will be free to download from Wednesday 20 January at www.nuffieldtrust.org.uk/publications

* The national averages for England are distorted by London, due to the capital's relatively young and healthy population, high labour costs and high concentration of teaching and research hospitals (which lower the crude productivity of its staff).

20 January 2010

⇨ The above information is reprinted with kind permission from The Nuffield Trust. Please visit www.nuffieldtrust.org.uk for more.

© *The Nuffield Trust*

NHS facing tough choices

Politicians must face reality of tough NHS financial future, says The King's Fund

Commenting in response to today's report from the NHS Confederation on the financial prospects for the NHS, The King's Fund's Chief Executive Niall Dickson said:

'After a decade of unprecedented spending, the NHS could face drastic cuts after 2011. This report backs up our analysis, which shows that the prospects for the NHS after 2011 will be severe unless the service responds now by improving efficiency and reforming the way care is delivered.

'Our analysis shows the NHS will probably have to operate under these much harsher financial conditions up to 2017 – yet at the same time more older people, more technology and higher expectations will create more demand for healthcare. We do have a window of opportunity – just under two years – when budgets still look relatively generous and the service can prepare for the lean years ahead.

'In practical terms that means every NHS organisation should be embarking on a rigorous programme of cost control, and every organisation should be working with others to redesign services to improve quality and save money. The two are not necessarily incompatible.

'But what is also required is political courage. We do not need politicians boasting that they will "spend more than the other lot" when they all know perfectly well that no matter who is in power the next few years will be about managing with less. This is not the time for reassurance – it is a time for difficult messages and support for doctors, nurses and managers who are prepared to reshape services at local level.

'That will mean driving efficiency throughout the system while focusing on the quality of care; concentrating some specialist services in fewer hospitals; moving other services into the community and learning to manage patients better to avoid unnecessary admissions and unnecessarily long stays in hospital. The alternative is to shy away from this agenda, pretend it will all be fine, and risk throwing away the significant advances that have been made in recent years.'

10 June 2009

⇨ The above information is reprinted with kind permission from The King's Fund. Visit www.kingsfund.org.uk for more information.

© *The King's Fund*

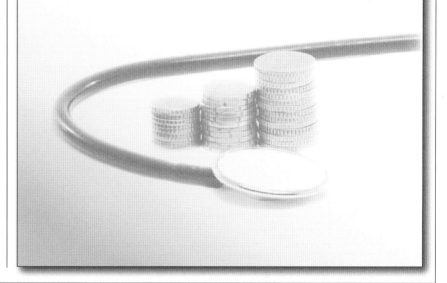

GP–patient relationship in need of first aid

Demos launches new report – *The Talking Cure: Why Conversation is the Future of Healthcare*

The conversation between GPs and patients – the cornerstone of modern healthcare in the UK – is under enormous pressure, and must be rethought for a less deferential age in which patients have access to vast amounts of medical information, a report launched today by Demos will argue.

> **The traditional model of 'doctor knows best' is being eroded. People, especially those with rare or chronic diseases, increasingly want to participate in their own treatments**

The report argues that the traditional model of 'doctor knows best' is being eroded. People, especially those with rare or chronic diseases, increasingly want to participate in their own treatments. GPs and policymakers must embrace patient engagement in medical treatment and healthcare, rather than stigmatising informed patients as 'cyberchondriacs'.

The pamphlet, produced in partnership with Pfizer UK, Rethink and Diabetes UK, and based on in-depth consultation with GPs, policy-makers and service users, argues that patient engagement can and should form the basis for effective health policy reform. Endless Whitehall quick-fixes only defer the problem; the real key to transforming the health system is to enable patients to actively participate in the conversations taking place in GP's consulting rooms.

Demos researcher and author of the study Jack Stilgoe said:

'Any GP will recognise the patient who comes into their surgery carrying armfuls of printouts from the Internet. But rather than groaning, doctors need to see this as a good thing. Patients are becoming experts too, and the NHS needs to acknowledge this and listen to them.

'As Lord Darzi puts the finishing touches to his review on the future of the NHS, the focus should be less about the mechanics of the system, and more about the people that are at the heart of healthcare.'

Report recommendations:

⇨ GPs and patients with chronic conditions should jointly establish 'outcome statements' with shared goals, creating a partnership between GP and patient;

⇨ Patients with long-term conditions should be allocated personal healthcare budgets to allow them to take part in building the services and care which suit them best;

⇨ Government should create 'Wiki-records' – online, accessible records which patients could contribute to and comment on;

⇨ Information and condition-specific 'patient packs' should be provided by GPs and the NHS as an integral part of treatment;

⇨ Patient groups such as Diabetes UK and Rethink should create pilot programmes to realise the vision of patient engagement set out by Derek Wanless in his 2002 report;

⇨ Government should place GP-patient relationships at the heart of the proposed NHS Constitution.

13 May 2008

⇨ The above information is reprinted with kind permission from Demos. Visit www.demos.co.uk for more information.

© Demos

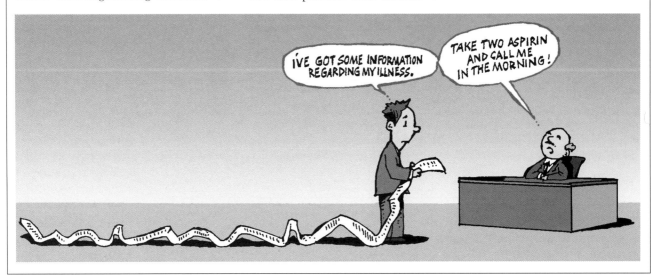

New legal rights for NHS patients

A consultation has been launched on legal rights to waiting times and NHS health checks for patients

Patients will have legal rights to maximum waiting times for elective procedures and urgent cancer referrals and to an NHS Health Check every five years for those aged 40-74, if proposals published today are taken forward.

The proposals, set out in *The NHS Constitution: A consultation on new patient rights*, will mean that from 1 April 2010, patients will have the legal right to maximum waiting times to start treatment by a consultant within 18 weeks of GP referral, and to be seen by a cancer specialist within two weeks of GP referral.

If the NHS is unable to meet this commitment, it will be required to take all reasonable steps to find a range of alternative providers that can. This will enable a patient to receive their care more quickly, if this is what they want. The alternatives could include private providers at NHS prices.

In addition, everyone aged 40-74 will have the right to an NHS Health Check every five years to assess their risk of heart disease, stroke, diabetes and kidney disease. Identifying any risk early should help to reduce the incidence of these diseases and the damage they cause.

Prime Minister Gordon Brown said:

'None of us can ever know what's around the corner and it's one of the best things about being British that the NHS will be there for us whatever happens. My own parents could never have afforded all the surgery needed to save my sight if they'd had to pay, and every day I hear from people whose lives have been saved or transformed by the NHS. Today we're reforming the NHS to secure its future – ensuring that patients get a guarantee not a gamble by empowering them with new legal rights.

'These measures build on the high standards and rightly rising expectations of patient care. Every single person who has to go into hospital or go through the difficulty of cancer will have clear rights and real power guaranteeing them quick access to care, or the offer of going private or to another NHS provider if these standards are not met.'

Health Secretary Andy Burnham said:

'The NHS Constitution lets people know what they can expect and what they can demand. But, like the NHS, the Constitution must evolve if it is to remain relevant.

'Waiting times are the shortest they have ever been but I want to build on this and give patients a legal right to maximum waiting times. Turning targets into legal rights will empower patients and guarantee them the same high standards of care, regardless of where they live.

'None of us can ever know what's around the corner and it's one of the best things about being British that the NHS will be there for us whatever happens'

'In the next decade, the NHS must make a decisive move towards being a more preventative service and a more people-centred service. So I want to give all patients aged 40-74 the legal right to have an NHS Health Check every five years. And we're also seeking views on whether there should be a legal right in future to choose to die at home and to personal health budgets to give people power over their own care.

'A decade of investment and reform has seen the NHS go from poor to good. Now, in striving to move from good to great we need to take a new

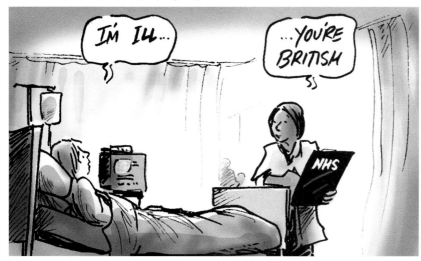

approach – less about central targets, more about rights and entitlements. These proposals will mean that patient rights, enshrined in the NHS Constitution, will safeguard the NHS for the future.'

Joe Korner, Director of Communications for The Stroke Association, said:

'We could save up to 40,000 people from having a stroke every year if we could make sure that their blood pressure and other risk factors for stroke were kept under control. That is why The Stroke Association believes these NHS Health Checks are so important.

'Stroke is the biggest cause of severe adult disability and the third biggest killer in the UK. NHS Health Checks will help to identify those at a higher risk of stroke and how to do something about it – whether that's through medication or taking steps to eat more healthily, get more exercise or give up smoking.'

Including these rights in the NHS Constitution would ensure that the NHS will never return to the days of patients waiting 18 months for treatment and offers people a quick and straightforward means of redress for the small number of cases where their rights are not met.

The consultation also seeks views on going even further and including more rights in the future. These could include:

⇨ the right to choose to die at home;
⇨ the right to access to NHS dentistry;
⇨ the right to personal health budgets;
⇨ the right to choose a GP practice offering extended access to evening and weekend appointments;
⇨ the right to key diagnostic tests for suspected cancer patients within one week of seeing a GP, with an interim milestone of two weeks.

10 November 2009

⇨ The above information is reprinted with kind permission from the Department of Health. Visit their website at www.dh.gov.uk for more information on this and other related topics.

© Crown copyright

Nurses to have degrees from 2013

Information from NHS Careers

The Government has announced that from 2013, all nurses will be educated to degree level. The proposal, which is supported by all the key national nursing bodies, is designed to make sure that new nurses are better equipped to improve the quality of patient care.

Nurses are the largest single profession within the NHS – there are currently around 400,000 nurses working in the NHS. They are critical to the delivery of high-quality healthcare. Nurses work in every sort of healthcare setting from accident and emergency to working in patients' homes, with people of all ages and backgrounds.

More young people than ever are studying for degree courses and the aim is that by becoming an all-degree profession, nursing will become more attractive to them.

Health minister Ann Keen MP commented:

'By bringing in degree level registration we can ensure new nurses have the best possible start to meet the challenges of tomorrow. Degree level education will provide new nurses with the decision-making skills they need to make high-level judgements in the transformed NHS.'

There are currently two main routes to becoming a nurse – either through a diploma course or a degree, with the main difference being that the degree course asks for higher academic entry requirements. However, diploma courses will be phased out between September 2011 and early 2013 and new entrants to the nursing profession from September 2013 will have to study a degree. This will not affect those studying for nursing diplomas in the next two years.

The Nursing and Midwifery Council, the profession's regulator, is developing new proposals for nurse education in line with the plan to provide all new nurses with degrees. They will consult widely with the public in early 2010 and announce the new standards and competencies later next year. It is expected that programmes at degree level using the new standards will start from September 2011.

Nurses work in an interesting, rewarding and challenging environment. If you are interested in working in a fast-paced, but above all caring, role then nursing may be for you. See our nursing pages for more information about the different types of nursing careers in the NHS and real-life stories of nurses currently working in the health service.

12 November 2009

⇨ The above information is reprinted with kind permission from NHS Careers. Visit www.nhscareers.nhs.uk for more information.

© NHS Careers

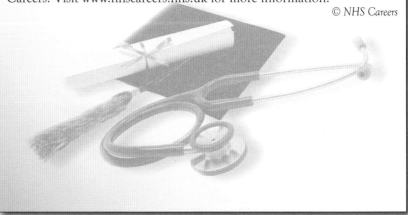

Undermining nursing care by degrees

The proposal that nurses in England should be university graduates will further reduce the level of basic nursing skills

Ann Keen, the health minister and a former nurse, wants to raise the status of nursing and the quality of patient care. Others, like the main nursing union, the Royal College of Nursing (RCN), and the chief nursing officer, Dame Chris Beasley, want to make nursing more attractive and to get rid of the stigma of nurses being 'doctors' handmaidens'. And the proposed solution to this problem that Keen plans to consult on? All newly qualified nurses should be university graduates by 2013, up from the current level of 25 per cent.

Admirable sentiments, considering how bad things have become, if a damning report published by the Patients Association this year is to be believed.[1] The report outlines the dreadful, neglectful, demeaning, painful and sometimes downright cruel treatment that patients and their elderly relatives have experienced at the hands of some National Health Service (NHS) nurses.

A row of sorts has erupted in response, suggesting that the problems identified will not be addressed by degree-based training. As a nurse of 35 years standing, I wholeheartedly agree.

By Brid Hehir

I believe that the most fundamental aspect of nursing – caring – has been degraded and devalued. Bedside care has been devolved to health care assistants with registered nurses undertaking more technical tasks. It's as if bedside care is no longer the remit of nurses.

But I don't think it's the role of universities to address this problem. Universities should not be used for instrumental purposes like teaching skills. Their role should be an entirely different one.

Nursing has been, and remains for many, a poorly paid occupation, although huge variations as well as opportunities exist within it. In the past, we were bought off with platitudes like nursing being a 'vocation' and being 'ministering angels', as if we were nuns, not health workers. Although we partially colluded with this patronising and demeaning view of ourselves, we at least felt, despite our lowly status, that we were doing the job for altruistic reasons. We felt valued, respected and trusted by patients and the public alike. We felt that we did a good, if hard, job, and gained a lot of satisfaction from helping people.

> **Universities should not be used for instrumental purposes like teaching skills. Their role should be an entirely different one**

Our professional organisations and trade unions didn't ever put up much of a fight to change our pay or conditions, however. Some even actively discouraged us from seeing ourselves as ordinary members of the public-sector workforce. We were supposed to be different. We cared, unlike the porters and domestic staff who took strike action from time to time. All that's changed, of course, as has the status of nurses – but not necessarily for the better in my estimation.

In wanting degree-based education for nurses, Keen and the RCN are presumably acknowledging that current nurse training is inadequate,

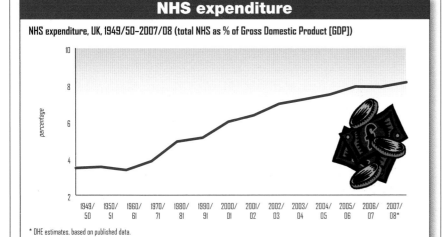

NHS expenditure

NHS expenditure, UK, 1949/50–2007/08 (total NHS as % of Gross Domestic Product (GDP))

* OHE estimates, based on published data.

Sources: Consumer Trends, Annual Abstract of Statistics, Economic Trends (Office for National Statistics); The Government's Expenditure Plans, Dept. of Health Departmental Report (Dept. of Health); NHS Board Operating Costs and Capital Expenditure, ISD Scotland (ISD); Public Expenditure Statistical Analyses (HM Treasury); Laing's Healthcare Market Review (Laing and Buisson); Population Projections Database (GAD); Health Statistics Wales (NAW).

at least as far as England is concerned. Nurse training in Wales is already degree-based. Prior to 1992, when diploma-level training was introduced, nurses spent only a quarter of their training in the classroom and three quarters on the wards. The supernumerary status that student nurses acquired in 1992 meant they were no longer part of the clinical workforce. They are now expected to learn through supervised participation – observing but not participating enough in the care that health care assistants and registered nurses perform.

It's not surprising, therefore, whether graduating with degrees or not, that many nurses qualify with quite basic and superficial knowledge and with nothing like enough skills, knowledge, clinical and practical experience. Much of this then has to be learnt after qualifying; the time when they should be consolidating what's been learnt, putting theory into practice and taking on new responsibilities and becoming good practitioners. Some never learn the skills adequately.

This invariably has a knock-on effect. Wards become staffed by poorly trained, inexperienced nurses not up to the job, who find basic nursing care challenging. The nurses who stick around and thrive, despite all of this, have to work under enormous pressure, trying to carry the load that their less-experienced colleagues can't share (and even add to), struggling to keep the show on the road and maintain standards and trying to ensure that patients are cared for competently and compassionately. Patient care is consequently sometimes less than adequate. And the pressure

this engenders contributes to many good nurses leaving the NHS.

But degree-level education is not the answer to the problem of inadequate training and poor care provision. Indeed, it may exacerbate it. As has been written about at length on *spiked*, degree-level education in Britain, in general, has long been inadequate and unchallenging for students and does many a disservice. It's even been suggested that a degree is now the equivalent of the school exam for 16-year-olds, the GCSE, because the standard has dropped so low.

But universities should not be teaching skills anyway. Instead, they should be helping students expand their minds, teaching them to think and to acquire knowledge for knowledge's sake. Leave skills training to the nursing colleges where it belongs.

The practical, attitudinal and compassionate skills that nurses need to acquire, so that they become intuitive in the provision of care, have to be learnt on the job. Theory ought to be after, not prior to actual experience. This practical side is the very aspect of training that nurses get an insufficient amount of already. The problem can only get worse if university-based training becomes the norm because the emphasis will shift further to theoretical aspects of caring as opposed to its practical application. That may well compound the existing prejudice about nurses being 'too posh to wash', delegating the work to less-qualified health care assistants.

These fundamental problems need to be acknowledged and discussed before going any further

with this consultation. Caring for sick people is a privilege and nurses need to be competent in providing it. When they are, their status will automatically improve. Nurses can and should be able to attend university after qualifying and when they've consolidated their knowledge and acquired the necessary nursing skills. Meanwhile Ann Keen and the RCN could review the seriously flawed 'Agenda for Change' they so enthusiastically support, to address the pay and conditions of nurses and other NHS staff.

Brid Hehir is head of engagement and patient involvement and sessional nurse in the NHS in London. She writes in a personal capacity.

Previously on *spiked*

Brid Hehir criticised the covert monitoring of NHS staff. Tim Black noted that the problem with degrees today was a society that has lost faith in learning. Dr Michael Fitzpatrick criticised the squalor of contemporary UK healthcare and argued that Darzi's interim report on the NHS profoundly misunderstood Britain's 'health crisis'. He also criticised the way Tony Blair alienated patients and degraded doctors. Brendan O'Neill declared we don't need any more patient choice.

Notes

1 *Patients not numbers, people not statistics*, Patients Association *17 November 2009*

⇨ The above information is reprinted with kind permission from *Spiked*. Visit www.spiked-online.com for more information.

© *Spiked*

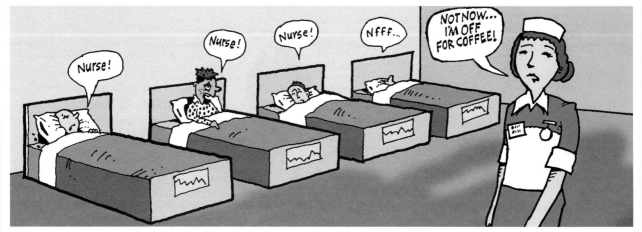

NHS 'could learn from John Lewis'

NHS could learn from John Lewis about motivating staff, says Nuffield Trust

Adopting principles from employee owned organis-ations, such as the major UK retail group the John Lewis Partnership, may help the NHS engage staff and deliver better services, says a report from The Nuffield Trust.

The Trust, which carries out research in healthcare services, looked at the international evidence on the effects of employee ownership on performance, including the operation of four such organisations: the John Lewis Partnership; Kaiser Permanente, a US healthcare provider; Circle, a European private healthcare provider; and Central Surrey Health, a provider of nursing and community healthcare services.

Employee-owned companies that allow staff to participate in making decisions on how the workplace is run can deliver a range of benefits

It found that employee-owned companies that allow staff to participate in making decisions on how the workplace is run can deliver a range of benefits, such as better productivity and performance, less staff turnover and sickness absence, greater innovation, and higher levels of motivation and commitment among the staff.

Although little research has looked at the effects of such participation on end users of services, some employee-owned organisations have a high degree of customer trust and loyalty, says the report.

By Zosia Kmietowicz

Chris Ham, professor of health policy and management at the University of Birmingham and one of the authors of the report, said that success in engaging NHS staff depends on their feeling valued and involved in decisions, but there was little evidence that this was happening.

He said, 'NHS staff are motivated by the opportunity to deliver high-quality services that make a difference to patients. But they feel that their ability to do this is being threatened by the adoption of a more business-oriented approach within the health service. The challenge for the NHS is to achieve closer alignment of the interests and goals of frontline line staff and the organisations that they work for.'

Last year's 'next stage review' of the NHS by the health minister Ara Darzi recognised the need for reforms of the NHS to be locally led and clinically driven and for greater freedoms for frontline staff. The NHS constitution, which is included in the health bill currently going through Parliament, also pledges that staff will be engaged in decisions that affect them and empowered to put forward ways of delivering better and safer services.

Jennifer Dixon, director of The Nuffield Trust, said that the Government was promoting new types of ownership in the NHS, such as social enterprises and foundation trusts, but that more needed to be done to help these develop.

Jo Ellins, of the Health Services Management Centre at the University of Birmingham and co-author of the report, said that two factors had to be present for employee-owned organisations to deliver benefits: 'managing staff in ways that foster their participation in the workplace and a culture of ownership that is associated with staff having a collective voice in the organisation'. *2 July 2009*

⇨ The above information is reprinted with kind permission from BMJ Publishing Group. Visit www.bmj.com for more information.

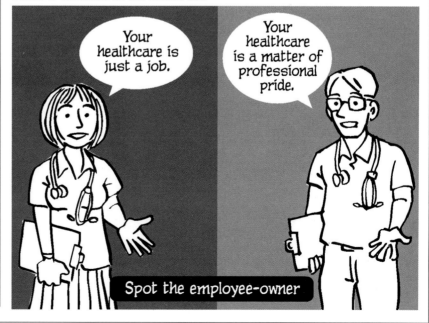

Your healthcare is just a job.

Your healthcare is a matter of professional pride.

Spot the employee-owner

An NHS strategy for a new era

Health Secretary Andy Burnham today set out his strategy for the NHS to put patients first and improve the quality of care as it enters an unprecedented era of reform

The strategy, 'NHS 2010–2015: from good to great. Preventative, people-centred, productive,' published today by the Department of Health, explains the need to accelerate the pace of NHS reform to make the system more productive and hasten improvements in quality of care – protecting patients, supporting staff, shifting resources to the frontline and slashing back office waste and bureaucracy.

> **'For the NHS to become truly great, it must become more preventative and people-centred'**

Andy Burnham said:

'The NHS today is better funded, more resilient, has more capacity and provides better care than ever before. It is ready to take on the new challenge of getting more out of what we have and moving from good to great.

'For the NHS to become truly great, it must become more preventative and people-centred. Lord Darzi's vision to put quality at the heart of the NHS is fast becoming a reality across the country. This means top quality care is our goal and patient safety our top priority. This is right for our times. Quality care is not always about spending more money, but about spending it in the right places. Moving care from hospitals into homes and communities is better for patients and more efficient.

'With an ageing population and the increased prevalence of lifestyle diseases, preventing illness and keeping people healthy is our best long-term insurance policy for the nation's health and managing the financial challenges ahead. The NHS should intervene earlier to help people lead healthier lives and prevent more disease.

'The improvements in the last decade have been made by NHS staff. It is vital to protect frontline staff in order to deliver services to patients. The challenge to the NHS, and to NHS leaders and staff around the country, is to reshape services further and faster than ever before. We are proud of the achievements of NHS staff and we will do everything we can to support them through the next period of change.

'In the past, a tougher financial environment has meant that patients have paid the price through longer waits. But that will not happen this time. We will not back away from the NHS. The Pre-Budget Report confirms that we can lock-in the achievements of the last decade, while protecting patients and providing top quality care.

'I have said that the NHS is our preferred provider. This is not about accepting under-performance or freezing out our partners in other parts of the NHS, the third sector and the independent sector. But we are asking the NHS and its staff to go through an unprecedented amount of change, so this is about saying that where there is under-performance and the NHS is an incumbent provider, we will give the NHS the first opportunity to improve to the level of the best.'

The measures include:

⇨ A new payment system, which puts patients first – hospital income will increasingly be linked to patient satisfaction, rising to ten per cent of their payments over time, meaning hospitals will work harder for their patients.

⇨ More choice for patients – abolishing GP practice boundaries, improving access to a GP in the evenings and weekends and more services at home or in the community.

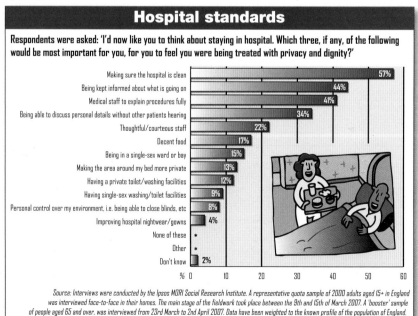

Hospital standards

Respondents were asked: 'I'd now like you to think about staying in hospital. Which three, if any, of the following would be most important for you, for you to feel you were being treated with privacy and dignity?'

	%
Making sure the hospital is clean	57%
Being kept informed about what is going on	44%
Medical staff to explain procedures fully	41%
Being able to discuss personal details without other patients hearing	34%
Thoughtful/courteous staff	22%
Decent food	17%
Being in a single-sex ward or bay	15%
Making the area around my bed more private	13%
Having a private toilet/washing facilities	12%
Having single-sex washing/toilet facilities	9%
Personal control over my environment, i.e. being able to close blinds, etc	8%
Improving hospital nightwear/gowns	4%
None of these	*
Other	*
Don't know	2%

Source: Interviews were conducted by the Ipsos MORI Social Research Institute. A representative quota sample of 2000 adults aged 15+ in England was interviewed face-to-face in their homes. The main stage of the fieldwork took place between the 9th and 15th of March 2007. A 'booster' sample of people aged 65 and over, was interviewed from 23rd March to 2nd April 2007. Data have been weighted to the known profile of the population of England.

- Dedicated carers for those in need: for patients with cancer or serious long-term conditions who can benefit from a more personal approach to nursing. Where appropriate, this should include the provision of personalised one-to-one support by a health professional, particularly for the more complex conditions.
- New rights to high-quality care including consulting on the right for patients nearing the end of their life to choose where they wish to spend their final days and new rights to high-quality standards of service and care that will be clearly set out in the new NHS Constitution.
- Supporting staff – we believe the announcement in the Pre-Budget Report provides the resources to protect frontline services in the NHS. We are proposing to work with NHS employers and trade unions through the national Social Partnership Forum and Staff Council to explore the pros and cons of whether we could offer frontline staff an employment guarantee locally or regionally – in return for flexibility, mobility and sustained pay restraint.
- More freedom for the best hospitals to expand their services out into the community across a wider area including GP centres.
- More access to personal care plans that allow patients to choose the right care tailored to their individual needs.
- Personal health budgets to empower patients; to give millions of patients the right to more control over their care and the services they can ask for, as well as more options to receive care at or closer to home.
- Locking in improvements in the service with the NHS Constitution – from 1 April 2010, we will give patients the legal right to maximum waiting times to start treatment by a consultant within 18 weeks of GP referral and to being seen by a cancer specialist within two weeks of GP referral. In addition, the Prime Minister announced in September plans to offer all patients in England access to tests that can confirm or exclude cancer within one week to help save thousands of lives every year.
- From April 2012, we also want everyone between 40 and 74 to have the legal right to an NHS Health Check every five years to assess their risk of heart disease, stroke, diabetes and kidney disease.
- Regular free health checks will improve health and prevent up to 1,600 heart attacks and strokes each year.

In addition, NHS Chief Executive David Nicholson today outlined details of the NHS Operating Framework for 2010/11, due to be published next week, which will set out NHS priorities for the next year. The Operating Framework will help the NHS make the changes necessary to embed quality and for it to drive all that the NHS does.

The Framework will allow the NHS to focus on ensuring care is safe, compassionate and personal to patients and will provide real opportunity for radical and innovative approaches to improve the quality of services, whilst at the same time reducing costs.

Notes

1 'NHS 2010-2015: from good to great. Preventative, people-centred, productive,' is available on the Department of Health website: www.dh.gov.uk

2 The top five priorities for the NHS in the Operating Framework remain:
- improving standards of cleanliness and tackling healthcare-associated infections;
- improving access to care through the achievement of the 18-week referral to treatment pledge and improving access to GP services, including at evenings and at weekends;
- improving the health of adults and children and reducing health inequalities, by focusing on improving care for cancer and stroke, and paying particular attention to children's health, especially in the most deprived areas of the country;
- improving patient experience, staff satisfaction and engagement; and
- preparing to respond in a state of emergency, such as an outbreak of pandemic influenza.

10 December 2009

- The above information is reprinted with kind permission from the Department of Health. Visit www.dh.gov.uk for more information on this and other related topics.

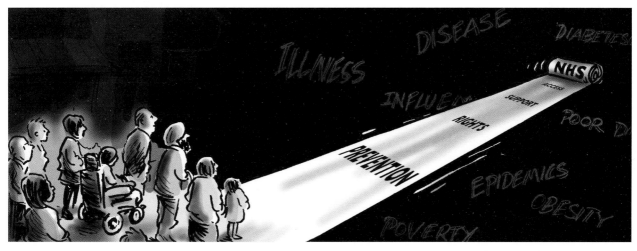

KEY FACTS

⇨ With the exception of charges for some prescriptions and optical and dental services, the NHS remains free at the point of use for anyone who is resident in the UK. That is currently more than 60 million people. (page 1)

⇨ The NHS currently employs 133,662 doctors, 408,160 qualified nursing staff, and 39,913 managers. (page 3)

⇨ The NHS deals with over a million patients every 36 hours. (page 4)

⇨ The National Health Service was established on 5 July 1948. For the first time hospitals, doctors, nurses, pharmacists and dentists provided services that were free for all at the point of delivery. (page 8)

⇨ Respondents to a Patients Association survey had concerns about spending on NHS bureaucracy. When asked what they considered a waste, nearly 30% believe non-clinical staff contribute to waste in the NHS. (page 11)

⇨ 44% of people surveyed by YouGov felt that 'a great deal of money' was being wasted in the NHS. (page 13)

⇨ Most patients are satisfied with the care they receive at their surgery (91%), including 56% who are very satisfied. Only four percent are dissatisfied. (page 16)

⇨ Most patients (81%) are satisfied with the opening hours of their surgery (including 43% who are very satisfied), but 54% would still like their surgery to open at additional times. (page 17)

⇨ Doctors have been named the profession most trusted by the general public for the 25th year running, according to the latest Ipsos MORI survey commissioned by the Royal College of Physicians. (page 18)

⇨ From January 2009, no one in England waits more than 18 weeks from the time they are referred to the start of their treatment. Most importantly, the average wait for treatment is much shorter, at just eight weeks. And median waiting times are just over two weeks for outpatients and four weeks for inpatients. (page 20)

⇨ NICE does not put a limit on the amount the NHS can spend on an individual patient. (page 21)

⇨ The government developed NICE to get rid of 'the postcode lottery' – where some drugs and treatments were available in some parts of the country, but not in others. NICE aims to give independent advice about which treatments should be available on the NHS in England and Wales. (page 22)

⇨ Giving people financial incentives to change their behaviour or adhere to medication regimens is becoming a more frequent approach adopted by healthcare providers around the world, often attracting controversy. (page 24)

⇨ The NHS is cheap by international standards. For example, the UK spent 7.1% of Gross Domestic Product (GDP) on health care in 2000, most of this on the NHS, while the average for the rest of the European Union (EU) in 1998 (latest data available) was 9.2%. (page 25)

⇨ Critics say that the NHS is not as efficient as it could be. Some hospitals need to be closed and the resources transferred into community health care. (page 26)

⇨ The number of death certificates in England and Wales mentioning Clostridium difficile or MRSA as a contributory factor fell sharply between 2007 and 2008. (page 29)

⇨ The Patients Association has said that devolution has led to a widening gap between NHS provision in England and the rest of the UK, with patients in Scotland, Wales and Northern Ireland getting a better deal. (page 29)

⇨ Nuffield Trust research suggests the NHS in England spends less and has fewer doctors, nurses and managers per head of population than the health services in the devolved countries, but that it is making better use of the resources it has in terms of delivering higher levels of activity, crude productivity of its staff and lower waiting times. (page 30)

⇨ The conversation between GPs and patients – the cornerstone of modern healthcare in the UK – is under enormous pressure, and must be rethought for a less deferential age in which patients have access to vast amounts of medical information, a report argues. (page 32)

⇨ The Government has announced that from 2013, all nurses will be educated to degree level. The proposal, which is supported by all the key national nursing bodies, is designed to make sure that new nurses are better equipped to improve the quality of patient care. (page 34)

⇨ Adopting principles from employee owned organisations, such as the major UK retail group the John Lewis Partnership, may help the NHS engage staff and deliver better services, says a report from the Nuffield Trust. (page 37)

⇨ 57% of respondents in an Ipsos MORI survey said that the most important thing for them to feel they were being treated with privacy and dignity during a stay in hospital would be making sure the hospital is clean. (page 37)

GLOSSARY

Devolved healthcare

When people refer to devolved healthcare, they are talking about the fact that NHS services, while funded centrally, are managed separately by the constituent countries of the UK: England, Wales, Scotland and Northern Ireland. There are therefore differences in how healthcare is provided in each country – for example, NHS users in Wales are able to get their prescriptions for free, while this is not the case in neighbouring England.

GP

GP stands for General Practitioner. This is a doctor who provides primary care: for example, a local or family doctor.

Matrons

Matrons were senior nurses responsible for supervising hospital wards. In the early days of the NHS, the matrons were very powerful figures in hospitals. They often had formidable reputations and were know for being very strict with patients and visitors, as well as adhering to rigorous hygiene standards. The stereotype of an intimidating hospital matron was popularised by the actress Hattie Jacques in films like *Carry On Doctor*.

Patients

Someone receiving medical treatment. An outpatient is someone who does not need an overnight stay in hospital as part of their treatment, while an inpatient will require a hospital bed for one night or more.

National Institute for health and Clinical Excellence (NICE)

NICE is an independent organisation set up by the Government in 1999 to try and eradicate the so-called 'postcode lottery', where some medicines and treatments were available in certain regions but not in others. NICE decides which drugs and treatments should be available on the NHS in England and Wales by assessing whether treatments will be cost-effective and beneficial to patients. Scotland and Northern Ireland have separate organisations to make decisions.

The NHS

The National Health Service (NHS) was launched in 1948, with the aim of providing healthcare funded by national taxation and free at the point of access for all UK residents – today, that is more than 60 million people. The NHS is one of the world's biggest employers and deals with one million patients every 36 hours. Although most people do not oppose the provision of free healthcare in the UK, some campaigners have drawn attention to problems in the NHS, such as poor hygiene standards in some hospitals, the degrading treatment of a minority of patients, 'postcode lotteries', long waiting lists for some treatments and financial waste.

Pharmaceutical companies

The pharmaceutical industry develops, produces and markets drugs licensed for use as medications.

Primary care trusts (PCTs)

PCTs provide care when you first have a health problem and need to visit a doctor. They work with local authorities and health and social care agencies, overseeing 29,000 GPs and 18,000 NHS dentists. There are 152 primary care trusts and they control 80 per cent of the NHS budget.

Private healthcare

While everyone in the UK has a right to free healthcare via the NHS, some people choose to pay out of their own pocket for private healthcare. This can be paid for through medical insurance, or on an ad hoc basis each time it is used. Some advantages of going private are: avoiding NHS waiting lists; getting medical treatment not available on the NHS, and having more comfortable accommodation. However, some illnesses or treatments covered by the NHS may not be covered by private medical insurance – for example, fertility treatment.

Superbugs

The term 'superbugs' refers to a group of hospital infections which are resistant to antibiotics. Outbreaks in hospitals are very dangerous, even lethal. The most well-known superbugs are MRSA and C. difficile.

INDEX

Additional Resources

Other Issues titles

If you are interested in researching further some of the issues raised in *Health and the State*, you may like to read the following titles in the **Issues** series:

➪ Vol. 176 *Health Issues for Young People* (ISBN 978 1 86168 500 1)

➪ Vol. 173 *Sexual Health* (ISBN 978 1 86168 487 5)

➪ Vol. 167 *Our Human Rights* (ISBN 978 1 86168 471 4)

➪ Vol. 164 *The AIDS Crisis* (ISBN 978 1 86168 468 4)

➪ Vol. 163 *Drugs in the UK* (ISBN 978 1 86168 456 1)

➪ Vol. 162 *Staying Fit* (ISBN 978 1 86168 455 4)

➪ Vol. 152 *Euthanasia and the Right to Die* (ISBN 978 1 86168 439 4)

➪ Vol. 145 *Smoking Trends* (ISBN 978 1 86168 411 0)

➪ Vol. 143 *Problem Drinking* (ISBN 978 1 86168 409 7)

➪ Vol. 141 *Mental Health* (ISBN 978 1 86168 407 3)

➪ Vol. 135 *Coping with Disability* (ISBN 978 1 86168 387 8)

➪ Vol. 81 *Alternative Therapies* (ISBN 978 1 86168 276 5)

For more information about these titles, visit our website at www.independence.co.uk/publicationslist

Useful organisations

You may find the websites of the following organisations useful for further research:

➪ **Demos:** www.demos.co.uk

➪ **Department of Health:** www.dh.gov.uk

➪ **Economic and Social Research Council:** www.socialscienceforschools.org.uk

➪ **Health Protection Agency:** www.hpa.org.uk

➪ **Ipsos MORI:** www.ipsos-mori.com

➪ **The King's Fund:** www.kingsfund.org.uk

➪ **NetDoctor:** www.netdoctor.co.uk

➪ **NHS Choices:** www.nhs.uk

➪ **NHS Confederation:** www.nhsconfed.org

➪ **The Nuffield Trust:** www.nuffieldtrust.org.uk

➪ **Office of Health Economics:** www.ohe.org

➪ **Patients Survey:** www.patients-association.org.uk

➪ **Royal College of Physicians:** www.rcplondon.ac.uk

➪ **TheSite:** www.thesite.org

➪ **UNISON:** www.unison.org.uk

➪ **Wellcome Trust:** www.wellcome.ac.uk

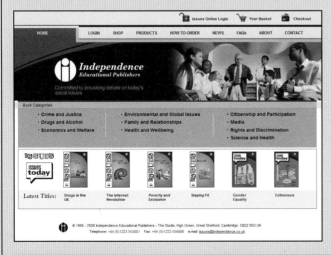
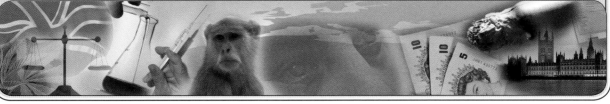

ACKNOWLEDGEMENTS

The publisher is grateful for permission to reproduce the following material.

While every care has been taken to trace and acknowledge copyright, the publisher tenders its apology for any accidental infringement or where copyright has proved untraceable. The publisher would be pleased to come to a suitable arrangement in any such case with the rightful owner.

Chapter One: The NHS
About the NHS – an overview, © Crown copyright is reproduced with the permission of Her Majesty's Stationery Office, Private healthcare, © TheSite.org, Key statistics on the NHS, © NHS Confederation, What is the NHS?, © NetDoctor, The changing health service, © ESRC, NHS 60 years on: snails, snow and Matron, © Telegraph Group Limited, London 2010, How healthy are we?, © Crown copyright is reproduced with the permission of Her Majesty's Stationery Office, The NHS at 60, © Patients Association, The NHS Constitution, © Crown copyright is reproduced with the permission of Her Majesty's Stationery Office, The GP patient survey 2009/10, © Ipsos MORI, Doctors once again most trusted profession, © Royal College of Physicians, 'Evil and Orwellian', © Guardian Newspapers Ltd 2010, Why we love the NHS, © UNISON, What is NICE and how does it work?, © Cancer Research UK, Should NHS offer incentives to improve health?, © Wellcome Trust.

Chapter Two: Healthcare Problems
Has the NHS been successful?, © OHE 2009 www.ohe.org, Patients not numbers, people not statistics, © Patients Association, Common hospital superbugs, © Telegraph Newspapers Ltd, London 2010, Fall in deaths linked to C. difficile and MRSA, © Crown copyright is reproduced with the permission of Her Majesty's Stationery Office, England is 'poor relation' of NHS devolution, © Guardian Newspapers Limited 2010, Devolved healthcare, © The Nuffield Trust, NHS facing tough choices, © The King's Fund, GP–patient relationship in need of first aid, © Demos.

Chapter Three: Healthcare Solutions
New legal rights for NHS patients, © Crown copyright is reproduced with the permission of Her Majesty's Stationery Office, Nurses to have degrees from 2013, © NHS Careers, Undermining nursing care by degrees, © Spiked, NHS 'could learn from John Lewis', © BMJ Publishing Group, An NHS strategy for a new era, © Crown copyright is reproduced with the permission of Her Majesty's Stationery Office.

Photographs
Stock Xchng: pages 4, 17 (Sanja Gjenero); 7 (Lysanne Ooteman); 12 (Tomasz Kobosz); 19 (Adam Ciesielski); 21 (Iwan Beijes); 24 (Carl Silver/Niels Timmer); 26 (Vangelis Thomaidis); 27 (Wojciech Wolak); 29 (whirlybird/sanja gjenero); 31 (Vangelis Thomaidis); 34 (Paul Barker/Mary Gober). Wikimedia Commons: page 28 (Owain.davies).

Illustrations
Pages 3, 18, 32, 36: Don Hatcher; pages 6, 20, 33, 39: Simon Kneebone; pages 9, 16, 25, 37: Angelo Madrid; pages 14, 22: Bev Aisbett.

And with thanks to the team: Mary Chapman, Sandra Dennis, Claire Owen and Jan Sunderland.

Lisa Firth
Cambridge
January, 2010